HANDBOOK OF CONTRACEPTION AND FAMILY PLANNING

HANDBOOK OF CONTRACEPTION AND FAMILY PLANNING

SUZANNE EVERETT

Clinical Nurse Specialist, Family Planning,
The Margaret Pyke Centre; and Research Nurse,
The Margaret Pyke Memorial Trust, London, UK

Baillière Tindall
An imprint of Harcourt Publishers Limited

❦ is a registered trademark of Harcourt Publishers Limited

This book is printed on acid-free paper

First published 1998
  Reprinted 2000

A catalogue record for this book is available from the British Library

ISBN 0–7020–2001–X

Typeset by Phoenix Photosetting, Chatham, Kent
Printed and bound in China

NPCC/02

Dedicated to Florence Skelton, Violet Phillips and Isobel Everett.

CONTENTS

INTRODUCTION

This book aims to offer a comprehensive introduction to the role of the family planning nurse. It addresses some of the problems encountered during consultations, and offers the opportunity to test and evaluate your knowledge through self assessment questions. The answers to these questions are discussed at the end of each chapter.

Family planning as a profession is constantly changing as new methods of contraception become available and as new research is published. All health professionals are accountable for their own actions, and as management procedures may vary from hospital trusts and GP practices, it is important that you regularly update and understand policies within your workplace, which may be different from this book. It is vital for professionals to keep their knowledge updated. There are several ways to ensure that this happens:

❖ By becoming a member of the RCN Family Planning Forum and the National Association of Nurses for Contraception and Sexual Health (NANCSH) who both produce newsletters and organise conferences.

❖ By undertaking psychosexual seminar work which involves reflecting on the nurse–client relationship. By looking at the feelings evoked in the nurse–client relationship in this way, problems encountered are seen from a new perspective, helping the nurse's approach to them in the future.

❖ By keeping a reflective diary (Benner, 1994) insight can be gained which may be unavailable if an area is new to a nurse, which can improve future nursing care.

THE CONSULTATION

During a consultation you are in a unique position to give men and women the opportunity to talk about intimate areas of their sexual life and anxieties they may have. However, this will only happen when a client feels they are free to discuss any anxiety or problem. Sometimes clients will give you clues of a problem as they have their handle on the door and are about to leave the room. Sometimes we miss these clues because we are in a rush or fail to recognise the significance of the clue and only realize its meaning on reflection. In some situations we may neglect a statement because we have become caught up in our own beliefs. Clients may tell you information about themselves which may be upsetting and shocking to you; if your body language, tone of voice or expression shows this then they will feel that they are unable to disclose any further information for fear of being reproached and judged. It is important never to assume that all clients are heterosexual: family planning is not just about preventing pregnancy, but about disease prevention, health promotion and education.

During a consultation, ensure that you are free of interruptions and that total privacy is maintained. Give clients the opportunity to ask questions. Try and ask open ended questions, for example 'do you ever have pain or any difficulties during sexual intercourse?' rather than a closed question such as 'you don't have any pain during intercourse?' which only offers the client the opportunity to say 'no'. Open ended questions give clients room to bring up problems associated with the area of questioning. Open ended questions can allow clients to express problems which may in fact be common place; sometimes clients can feel that they are the only one having difficulties with, for example, a method of contraception, and knowing that they are not alone can be reassuring.

When undertaking any procedure involving a client, it is important to obtain their consent. For a client to give informed consent you should explain carefully why this procedure is necessary and what it involves. When performing intimate examinations such as vaginal or breast examinations, you should maintain the client's privacy, allowing them to feel safe without fear of being interrupted by your colleagues or viewed from windows by strangers.

If you give clients freedom to talk in a non-judgmental environment, then even if they choose not to disclose a problem at an initial consultation, they may return in the future knowing they can feel safe to talk freely.

HISTORY TAKING

At initial consultations with clients, a full medical history should be taken and updated at regular intervals, which must be dated and documented in the notes for future reference. A complete history includes the general health of the client in the past and present, their gynaecological and sexual health, contraceptive history, and the health of their immediate family. Clients can feel threatened by personal questions, especially if they are asked immediately on arrival; try and establish a rapport by finding out the reason for their attendance. Often by finding out why a client is attending, other questions that you need to know will be answered as a by-product. However, you will need to ask questions which should be open ended such as 'do you ever have any pre-menstrual symptoms?' or 'do you ever have migraines?' If a client does have a problem then you will need to find out more details: for example, if a client has migraines ask her to describe them and the frequency. You will still need to ask specific questions to eliminate contraindications to different methods of contraception such as 'when you have a migraine do you ever see flashing lights or have loss of vision?' Taking a detailed history can take time but can help nurture a good relationship between you and your client. It can also create the opportunity for them to discuss issues for which insufficient time was given previously.

THE CLIENT

Clients who attend for advice on family planning can vary not only in the cultural and religious beliefs they hold, but can also have very different attitudes and values about relationships and sexuality. The decisions and problems a client will encounter will depend on where they are in their life: for example, an unplanned pregnancy may be a disaster to a client aged either 15 or 50 for very different reasons, and the decision they make about the pregnancy will be from different perspectives.

Clients who are under 16 years of age may have taken some time to gain enough courage to attend a family planning clinic, and as a result may feel embarrassed and awkward. Often younger clients may attend with a friend and there may be anxiety over confidentiality, especially if the client is under the age of 16 (see confidentiality page 173). They may have already commenced sexual intercourse and require emergency contraception or already be pregnant. Research (Smith, 1993) has shown that the teenage pregnancy rate is higher in deprived areas, but the abortion rate is higher in affluent areas. The abortion rate may be higher in affluent areas for a number of reasons such as social and parental pressure, or that girls from these areas may know how to access abortion services and have the support of their parents. They may have career plans and see a future ahead (Simms, 1993), whilst teenagers living in deprived areas may decide to continue with a pregnancy because of lack of access to abortion services. They may not have career plans and see a pregnancy as their future.

Older clients may feel just as awkward as younger clients but for different reasons. They may not have discussed intimate areas of their sexual life with anyone, and may find the situation embarrassing. Society tends to portray clients over the age of 65 as disinterested in sexual intercourse; however, research shows this is far from the truth (Steinke, 1994). Nevertheless, with increasing age clients may need to adapt their sexual relationship depending on their health, and may wish to discuss this. Often the impact of chronic diseases and medications on sexuality are not fully discussed with clients and their partners. It may take clients some time before they are able to pluck up the courage to discuss these implications, or are given the opportunity by professionals to discuss them.

THE NURSE–CLIENT RELATIONSHIP

During a consultation a relationship develops between the nurse and the client where feelings and emotions may be expressed. Many clients who consult have no problems and attend for contraceptive advice and supplies; however, other clients may have anxieties and problems which take a great deal of courage to discuss. It is during consultations where there are problems that the recognition of feelings evident within the consultation can help illuminate these problems. This can be sufficient to relieve an anxiety or may bring a hidden problem out into the open, where it can be looked at more closely.

Recognising the type of emotion expressed in a consultation can be difficult, and sometimes you may only be able to recognise on reflection once a client has left. Reflection and psychosexual seminar training can help improve and increase your skills in this area. There are several reasons why we may fail to recognise feelings or acknowledge a problem. Sometimes we lack the confidence to discuss intimate areas with clients, and need a great deal of courage to pursue an issue, but this does become easier with practice. On other occasions our minds may be fixed on our own agenda which will stop us from listening to the client. For example there may be a very busy clinic and you may feel pressurised to 'hurry things along' or something the client says may trigger a memory or anxiety in your own personal life. You may have a strong desire 'to make things better for the client'. However, listening and being there for them is actually what they want, and learning to do this can be difficult initially. There may be occasions when you feel you are not establishing a relationship with the client and are unsure why this is so.

There are several ways to improve your skills in your relationship with your client:

❖ Practice listening and recalling conversations. Careful listening can help us pick up clues about how the client feels. Listening will also give you information about the client, which you will need to refer back to as clients will notice very quickly if you are not listening to what they are talking about.

❖ Learn to observe the body language of your clients. You can practice this by watching people around you.

❖ What is the client not saying, what are the feelings you are picking up through her body language, tone of voice, facial expression?

❖ By undertaking Balint seminar training. This is where a group of nurses meet for a set period of time with a seminar leader to discuss the nurse's work. As a group they listen and focus on the feelings invoked by the work; this helps the nurse to look at their work from a new perspective.

❖ Further education like the advanced family planning course ENB A08 can improve your skills and also increase knowledge in family planning.

❖ Lastly a personal reflective diary of your work can help improve your skills.

CONFIDENTIALITY AND ETHICS

All clients have the right to expect that information about themselves or others which is divulged during a consultation will remain confidential. Confidentiality should be respected and only broken in exceptional situations such as if the health, welfare, or safety of someone other than the client is at serious risk. If possible, clients should be sensitively encouraged to discuss exceptional areas with people involved themselves. Doctors/nurses who breach confidentiality must be able to show good reason for making this decision (UKCC, 1996), which would be a ethical decision. Ethics are the moral code by which a nurse's behaviour is governed within their work with clients and their families and the colleagues they work with.

Clients under the age of 16 are often concerned that any disclosures about their sexual life will be divulged to their parents. This can prevent clients from seeking help with contraception, resulting in unprotected sexual intercourse. Following the Gillick case, the House of Lords (BMA/GMSC/HEA/Brook Advisory Centres/FPA/RCGP, 1993) established that people under the age of 16 are able to give consent to medical treatment regardless of age, if they are able to understand what is proposed and the implications and consequences of the treatment. When clients under the age of 16 consult, doctors or nurses should consider the following issues:

❖ Whether the client understands the treatment, its implications and the risks and benefits of it.

❖ Health care professionals should encourage young clients to discuss their consultation with their parents, and their reasons for not wanting to do this. However, confidentiality will still be respected.

❖ Professionals should consider whether clients are likely to have sexual intercourse without contraception. They should also consider whether the mental and physical health of the client would suffer if the client was not to receive contraception. Lastly, it is important that the client's best interests are taken into account which may mean giving contraception and advice without parental consent.

Following the Data Protection Act 1984 and Access to Health Records Act 1990, clients have the right to have access to their written and computerized records. Where a client is under the age of 16 they may have access to their records if they are able to show an understanding of the reason for the application (Belfield, 1997). If a parent or guardian wishes to have access to these records this will not be permitted unless the client gives consent. If by giving a client access to their records another person's confidentiality would be breached then information to the other person should be withheld.

It is useful to think about these areas of confidentiality as clients (especially young clients) will often be concerned about this area, and you will need to be able to respond to this anxiety sensitively.

REFERENCES

Belfield T. (1997) FPA Contraceptive Handbook, 2nd edition. London: Family Planning Association (FPA).

Benner, P. (1994) From novice to expert. Menlo Park, California: Addison-Wesley.

BMA, GMSC, HEA, Brook Advisory Centres, FPA & RCGP (1993) Joint guidance note: *confidentiality and people under 16*. British Medical Association, General Medical Science Committee, Health Education Authority, Brook Advisory Centres, Family Planning Association and Royal College of General Practitioners.

Simms, M. (1993) Teenage pregnancy – give girls a motive for avoiding it. *British Medical Journal* **306:** 1749–1750 (letter).

Smith, T. (1993) Influence of socio economic factors on attaining targets for reducing teenage pregnancies. *British Medical Journal* **306:** 1232–1235.

Steinke, E. (1994) Knowledge and attitudes of older adults about sexuality in ageing: a comparison of two studies. *Journal of Advanced Nursing* **19:** 477–485.

UKCC (United Kingdom Central Council for Nursing, Midwifery and Health Visiting (1996) Guidelines for professional practice. London. UKCC.30.

ACKNOWLEDGEMENTS

No book is ever written by one person, without the help and support of other people. I would very much like to thank my colleagues Juliet Johnson, research nurse for The Margaret Pyke Trust, and Mary Hawkins, Clinical Nurse Specialist, for their support and help throughout this book, and the staff of The Margaret Pyke Trust and The Margaret Pyke Centre for their encouragement. I would also like to thank Jane Urwin, medical information officer at the Family Planning Association.

Many thanks to Ciara O'Rourke of Munro and Forster for providing slides and information on Norplant. Also thanks to Rosemary Hennings of Motech SAM for providing slides of Topaz and Becky Tam of Unipath for slides on Persona.

I would like to thank for her endless support Catriona Sutherland, Practice Nurse and Clinical Nurse Specialist, for reading through passages, giving advice and to her and Norman Sutherland for their support. Without the encouragement of my husband Jon through some pretty difficult times along with my parents, Graeme and Jenny, Cathy Doyle and Anne Taylor there definitely would not be a book.

Finally, I would like to thank Sarah James and Karen Gilmour of Baillière Tindall for their endless patience, support and for believing in me in the first place!

THE ANATOMY AND PHYSIOLOGY OF REPRODUCTION

I

INTRODUCTION

Reproductive biology is the science of the transmission of life. Just as with other animals, it is essential that humans reproduce in order to ensure the survival of their species.

The function of the reproductive system is to produce gametes (germ cells) and to provide the optimum conditions for the fusion of two gametes, one from the male and one from the female. The human female also has to provide a life-support system for the first 9 months of a new individual's life; thus her body must adapt and provide a suitable environment during that time.

THE FORMATION OF GAMETES

Before discussing the male and female reproductive systems in detail, it seems appropriate to consider meiosis, the process of cell division by which gametes are formed, and the factors that determine the genetic sex and phenotype (i.e. physical characteristics) of an individual.

THE DETERMINATION OF THE SEX OF AN INDIVIDUAL

In each human somatic cell there are 46 chromosomes, that is, 23 pairs. These are divided up into 22 pairs of autosomes and 1 pair of sex chromosomes; the latter are given the names X and Y due to the shape of the chromosomes. The human female has the complement XX in all her cells and the male XY in all his cells.

For each mating there is, in theory, a 50% chance (two out of four) that a female will result and a 50% chance that a male will result (Fig. 1.1). However, the observed sex ratio at birth shows that usually more males are born than females. The exact ratio varies from place to place and from time to time but, at present, in England and Wales the ratio at birth is approximately 106 males to every 100 females. It is not known what factor or factors favour conception by Y spermatozoa (for further reading see Parkes, 1976).

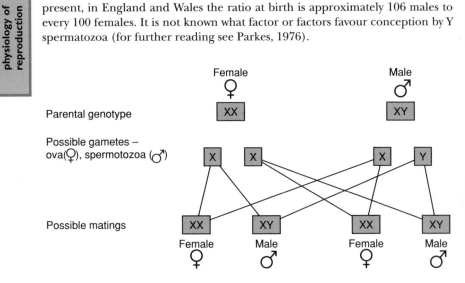

Fig. 1.1 Diagram showing the mechanism by which the chromosomal sex of an individual is determined.

However, more than the sex chromosome complement is involved in the determination of the gender of an individual. For example, for an individual to be truly male he needs an XY chromosome complement, normal male gonads (testes) and genitalia and the presence of normal quantities of male hormones. True females need an XX chromosome complement, normal female gonads (ovaries) and genitalia and the presence of normal quantities of female hormones.

THE FUNCTIONING OF THE MALE REPRODUCTIVE SYSTEM

A discussion of male reproductive physiology can be divided into three sections: the production of spermatozoa (the male gametes), the endocrine function of the testis, and the endocrine control of these processes. A brief description of the male reproductive system will be given first.

The male genital system consists of two testes and their ducts, several accessory glands and the penis (Fig. 1.2). The **testes** are situated in the scrotum. The tubules and ducts from each testis unite to form the **epididymis** (Fig. 1.3) and from here the **vas deferens** (ductus deferens) travels up into the pelvis, passes

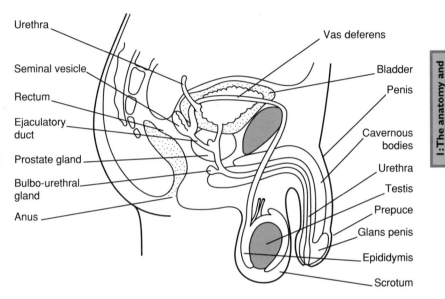

Fig. 1.2 Anatomy of the male reproductive system. The scrotum, penis and pelvic regions have been cut sagittally to show their internal structures.

anterior to the pubic symphysis and then loops around the ureter. At this point the vas deferens enlarges to become the ampulla. A **seminal vesicle**, one of the accessory sex glands, joins each vas at the lower end of the ampulla. The duct is then known as the **ejaculatory duct**. The two ejaculatory ducts (one from each ampulla and testis) fuse with the urethra in the middle of the prostate gland. The resultant duct, known as the **prostatic urethra**, is a common duct for both urination and the carriage of semen. The ducts from two additional accessory glands, the **bulbo-urethral glands** (Cowper's glands), join the urethra which enters the penis.

The **penis** is an elongated organ composed of mainly vascular spaces making up the erectile tissue and consists of three cylindrical bodies: two dorsal corpora cavernosa and ventrally one corpus spongiosum (Fig. 1.4). The penile urethra, which is lined with mucus-secreting glands, traverses the corpus spongiosum to the external urethral meatus. The head, or **glans penis**, is usually covered by the **prepuce**, or foreskin. Circumcision is the removal of the prepuce. If the prepuce is retracted for a long period of time, a paraphimosis may develop which involves constriction and swelling of the glans and an inability to restore it to the natural position.

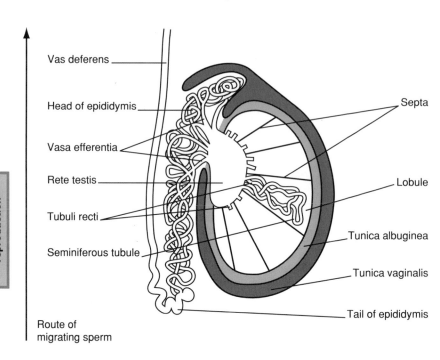

Vas deferens

Head of epididymis

Vasa efferentia

Rete testis

Tubuli recti

Seminiferous tubule

Route of migrating sperm

Septa

Lobule

Tunica albuginea

Tunica vaginalis

Tail of epididymis

Fig. 1.3 Structure of one testis.

Spermatogenesis

The production of spermatozoa, or spermatogenesis, occurs in the seminiferous tubules of the testis (see Fig. 1.3). Each testis is divided into many compartments, each containing one or more minute **seminiferous tubules**. Within each testicular compartment, connective tissue containing the **Leydig cells** (or **interstitial cells**) surrounds the seminiferous tubules. The Leydig cells are concerned with the synthesis and release of androgenic (male) hormones.

There are two types of cell in the seminiferous tubule of an active testis: the germ cells and the Sertoli cells. At any one time the germ cells are at various stages of development, but they all originate from **spermatogonia**. The spermatogonia undergo continuous mitotic divisions to ensure a constant supply of germ cells. Some of these cells mature and increase in size to become primary **spermatocytes**. These primary spermatocytes undergo the first meiotic division to become secondary spermatocytes, which then contain only the haploid number of chromosomes. The secondary spermatocytes undergo the second division of meiosis to become **spermatids**.

The spermatids are in close association with the Sertoli cells. The **Sertoli cells** are polymorphic cells (occurring in many shapes) that are attached to the basement membrane but extend into the lumen of the seminiferous tubule. The exact role of the Sertoli cells is unclear, but they are probably involved in the nutrition and support of the developing germ cells and may have some phagocytic action and endocrine influences.

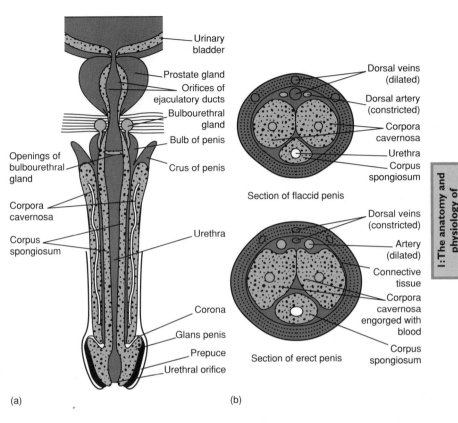

Fig. 1.4 Internal structure of the penis. (a) Longitudinal section through prostate gland and penis; (b) cross-section through flaccid and erect penis. Note that the erectile tissues of the corpora cavernosa and corpus spongiosum are engorged with blood in the erect penis.

The spermatids, still in close association with the Sertoli cells, undergo transformation from relatively simple cells into the highly specialized **spermatozoa**. Changes occur in both the nucleus and cytoplasm of the cell. The chromatin of the nucleus condenses to become the head of the spermatozoon; the Golgi apparatus contributes towards the formation of the **acrosome** (which contains hyaluronidases and proteinases that help the spermatozoon penetrate both the mucus plug of the cervix and the ovum); one of the centrioles in the cell lengthens to form the tail, and the mitochondria aggregate in the middle section of the spermatozoon. Any superfluous cytoplasm is lost (Fig. 1.5).

Once the spermatozoa have been produced, they are released from the Sertoli cells into the lumen of the seminiferous tubule. However, they are not functionally mature at this stage; completion of the maturation process occurs while the spermatozoa are stored in the epididymis. The total time taken for the production of mature spermatozoa from spermatogonia is approximately 70–100 days.

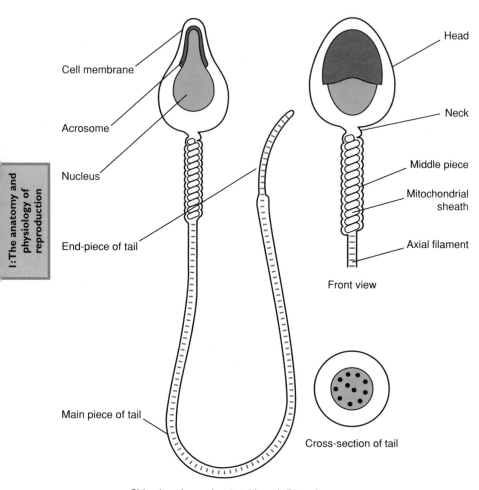

Cell membrane

Acrosome

Nucleus

End-piece of tail

Head

Neck

Middle piece

Mitochondrial
sheath

Axial filament

Front view

Main piece of tail

Cross-section of tail

Side view, in section (total length 50 µm)

Fig. 1.5 Structure of the mature spermatozoon.

Once fully formed, the spermatozoa are pushed out of the seminiferous tubules along the tubuli recti and into the rete testis and then via the vasa efferentia into the head of the epididymis (see Figs 1.3, 1.6). The **epididymis** is a long, coiled tube (if unravelled it would be approximately 6 m long) and is divided into sections – the head, body and tail – all closely applied to the posterior surface of the testis. The cilia in the tubuli recti beat and the smooth muscle around the tubules contracts, moving the spermatozoa towards the epididymis.

The time spent by the spermatozoa in the epididymis is an organized delay: it allows them to mature before ejaculation. It is thought that the secretory columnar epithelium of the epididymis secretes hormones, enzymes and nutrients that may be important for sperm maturation. The growth of the

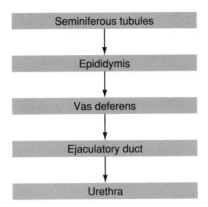

Fig. 1.6 **Route followed by spermatozoa from synthesis to ejaculation.**

epithelium of the epididymis is dependent on adequate levels of male sex hormones.

The tail of the epididymis is the main storehouse for the spermatozoa, although some may be stored in the vas. Storage is necessary because spermatogenesis is a continuous process, whereas ejaculation occurs at irregular intervals. If no ejaculation occurs, the spermatozoa in the epididymis ultimately degenerate and undergo liquefaction. It is also thought that the epithelial cells of the ducts may have phagocytic properties and may be able to remove abnormal spermatozoa. The spermatozoa mature in their abilities both to move and to fertilize ova during the passage through the excretory ducts, but the exact nature of this maturation process is not known. Spermatozoa can be stored in the genital ducts for as long as 42 days.

The vas deferens (or ductus deferens) is a muscular tube that begins in the scrotum as a continuation of the tail of the epididymis and ends in the pelvis by joining with the duct of the seminal vesicle in the formation of the ejaculatory duct. It ascends from the scrotum in the spermatic cord. The **spermatic cord** also contains blood vessels and nerves that supply the testes and also muscular and connective tissue extensions from the anterior abdominal wall.

The wall of the vas deferens is composed of an outer layer of loose connective tissue and three layers of smooth muscle with an abundant autonomic nerve supply. This arrangement accounts for the ability of the vas to contract quickly and efficiently during ejaculation. In addition to these peristaltic contractions, the spermatozoa are able to 'swim' by means of two-dimensional bending waves which pass from the front to the back end of their tails. The tails of the spermatozoa are composed of a central filament containing a pair of microfibrils surrounded by a circle of nine fibrils.

The role of the accessory sex glands

The accessory sex glands provide a transport medium, with the necessary nutrients, for the spermatozoa to leave the male and enter the female.

The seminal vesicles

These two glands are so called because they were originally thought to store the spermatozoa, but that is not their function; they are secretory glands. They are located behind the prostate gland and lateral to each ampulla of vas. Each vesicle is a muscular convoluted tube lined by secretory epithelium with a maximum capacity of 3 ml.

The secretion of the seminal vesicles is an alkaline, viscid, yellowish fluid containing, amongst other compounds, fructose, globulin, ascorbic acid and prostaglandins. It forms the fluid vehicle for the spermatozoa. Its secretory activity is under the control of the testicular hormones and in old age the vesicles diminish in size because of decreased hormone stimulation.

The prostate gland

The prostate gland is situated around the bladder neck and the first part of the urethra, into which its secretions pass. Its actual size varies considerably. At puberty the prostate gland increases rapidly in size and in the normal adult its shape is likened to a chestnut with an approximate 3 cm diameter in all directions; it remains fairly constant in size until middle age when it may involute or, more often, undergo benign hypertrophy which frequently results in urological problems. The main glandular tissue is situated in the lateral and posterior portions (known as the outer zone) of the prostate, whereas the inner zone (the middle of the gland) consists mainly of mucosal glands.

The **prostatic secretion** consists of a thin, slightly acidic, milky fluid containing enzymes, for example acid hydrolase, acid phosphatase, protease and fibrinolysin; it is also rich in calcium and citrates. It is responsible for the characteristic odour of semen. Prostatic secretion is thought to stimulate the motility of the spermatozoa, coagulate the fluid from the seminal vesicles and go some way towards neutralizing the prevailing vaginal acidity. As with the secretions of the seminal vesicles, prostatic secretory activity is dependent upon adequate stimulation by the testicular hormones. Any reduction of this stimulus results in involution of the gland and its secretory elements.

The bulbo-urethral glands

The bulbo-urethral, or Cowper's, glands are small globular glands and are roughly pea sized. They lie between the lower prostate and the penis, and their ducts open into the urethra. They secrete mucus which serves as a lubricant prior to ejaculation.

The composition of semen

Semen, or seminal fluid, consists of spermatozoa, the secretions of the genital tract, especially the epididymis, and the secretions of the associated accessory glands. The bulk of the semen (approximately 60%) originates from the seminal vesicles. The pH of the combined secretions is slightly alkaline (pH 7.2–7.4), the acid prostatic secretions being neutralized by the other components. The pH of semen is important because spermatozoa are rapidly immobilized in an acid medium. The pH of the vaginal secretions is acid (approximately pH 4.5) and the alkaline semen neutralizes the inhibitory effect of the acid vagina. Semen is also rich in hyaluronidase, an enzyme which causes breakdown of mucopolysaccharides and which facilitates passage through the cervical mucus and the chemicals surrounding the ovum.

The average volume of ejaculate is 3 ml (range of 2–6 ml) and contains approximately 300 million spermatozoa.

The number, morphology and motility of the spermatozoa give an indication of the fertility of the male and are used clinically in the assessment of infertility. The normal is considered to be:

❖ volume of ejaculate 2–6 ml

❖ density of spermatozoa 60–150 million ml^{-1}

❖ morphology 60–80% normal shape

❖ motility 50% should be motile after incubation for 1 hour at 37°C

A specimen of semen for investigation is obtained by masturbation. The volume and density will depend on the previous period of abstinence from sexual intercourse: frequent ejaculations lead to a progressive reduction in the spermatozoa count in the semen. Values outside these normal ranges may be an indication of infertility.

Spermatozoa may be stored at −70°C for weeks or even months, and their motility and fertilizing ability reappear when unfrozen. This property is sometimes used when specimens are used for artificial insemination either by husband or donor.

Sperm from men undergoing chemotherapy for cancer may also be stored, because infertility may sometimes result from the treatment.

The endocrine function of the testis

The testes are responsible for spermatogenesis, as already discussed, but they also function as an endocrine gland. The interstitial cells of Leydig synthesize, store and secrete androgens, principally testosterone. Very small quantities of oestrogens are also produced but their role, in the male, is obscure. Approximately 95% of the androgen is produced in the testis and the remainder in the adrenal glands.

Testosterone

Testosterone is a steroid molecule synthesized from cholesterol. Total plasma levels of testosterone in the adult male are 12–30 nmol l^{-1} (in the adult female the testosterone level is 0.5–2.0 nmol l^{-1}, of adrenal origin). Most of the testosterone is loosely bound with plasma proteins once it is released into the blood; it circulates in the plasma before becoming fixed to the target tissues and then it is finally metabolized and excreted by the liver.

Testosterone has widespread effects on the body, both on the reproductive organs and on the somatic tissues. Most of the effects of testosterone (and other androgens) can be directly related to the fact that it is an important anabolic agent, synthesizing complex molecules from simpler ones. Once in the cells, testosterone stimulates an increase in the synthesis of proteins; it probably directly influences the DNA and RNA in the cell. Its major functions are as follows:

❖ development of male physique

❖ stimulation of epiphyseal growth

❖ growth of facial and body hair

❖ lowering pitch of voice

❖ increased sebum secretion (skin)

❖ mild electrolyte retention (kidneys)

❖ development of libido.

The endocrine control of the male reproductive system

There are three levels of hormones involved in the control of the male reproductive system: namely, hypothalamic hormone, anterior pituitary hormones, and testicular hormones. Both spermatogenesis and androgen production are controlled by the anterior pituitary hormones, the gonadotrophins, namely **follicle-stimulating hormone** (FSH) and **luteinizing hormone** (LH). The latter is also known as **interstitial cell-stimulating hormone** (ICSH) in the male. FSH acts primarily on the seminiferous tubules as a stimulus for spermatogenesis. Small quantities of LH are also required, however, for the completion of spermatogenesis. LH, or ICSH, as this alternative name indicates, stimulates the production of androgen from the interstitial cells of Leydig.

The release of these gonadotrophins is in response to a stimulus from the hypothalamus, and the release of both FSH and LH appears to be controlled by one hypothalamic releasing hormone known as **gonadotrophin-releasing hormone (GnRH)**. It is also known as follicle-stimulating hormone/luteinizing hormone-releasing hormone (FSH/LH-RH) or simply LHRH.

The exact nature of the feedback control system is still uncertain but it involves a negative feedback acting at either or both hypothalamic and pituitary levels. If a male is castrated, that is, has his testes removed, there is a marked increase in the levels of plasma gonadotrophins. This suggests that there is normally some negative feedback, and it is thought that testosterone levels are one of the stimuli involved; for example, relatively high levels of testosterone exert an inhibitory effect on the hypothalamus (and possibly the anterior pituitary), reducing the release of GnRH (and FSH and LH).

Inhibin, a protein hormone, has been isolated from testicular extracts and this appears to inhibit FSH secretion. It is probable that inhibin is produced from the Sertoli cells in response to stimulation by FSH, and it then exerts a negative feedback on FSH release. Oestrogens secreted by the testes could also be involved in the negative feedback process (de Jong, 1987).

THE FUNCTIONING OF THE FEMALE REPRODUCTIVE SYSTEM

The discussion of female reproductive physiology will be divided into the following sections: the production of ova (the female gametes) and ovulation; the menstrual cycle and its relationship with ovulation; and finally, the events leading to fertilization and a brief review of pregnancy.

The anatomy of the female reproductive system is shown in Figs 1.7–1.9.

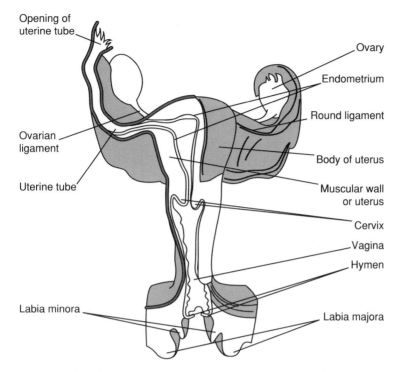

Opening of uterine tube

Ovary

Endometrium

Round ligament

Ovarian ligament

Body of uterus

Uterine tube

Muscular wall or uterus

Cervix

Vagina

Hymen

Labia minora

Labia majora

Fig. 1.7 Anterior view of the female reproductive system with some structures cut open to expose internal structure.

1: The anatomy and physiology of reproduction

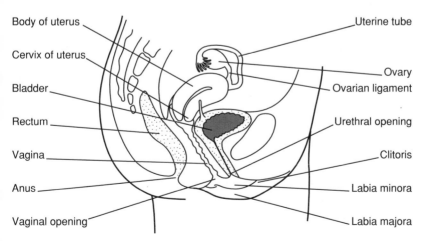

Body of uterus

Cervix of uterus

Bladder

Rectum

Vagina

Anus

Vaginal opening

Uterine tube

Ovary

Ovarian ligament

Urethral opening

Clitoris

Labia minora

Labia majora

Fig. 1.8 Median sagittal section of the female pelvis.

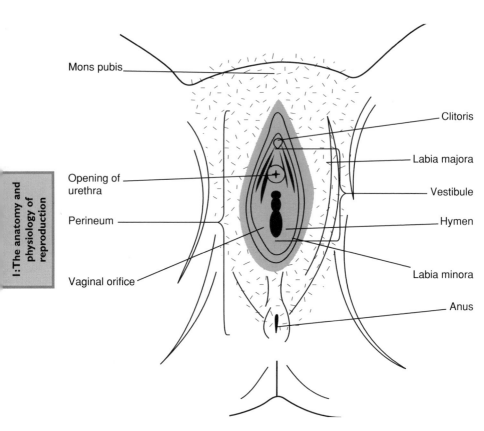

Fig. 1.9 The vulva.

Oogenesis and the ovarian cycle

The production of ova, or **oogenesis**, occurs in the ovaries. The **ovaries** vary in size and appearance according to the age of the female and the stage of the reproductive cycle. In the adult they are approximately 4 cm long, 2 cm wide and 1 cm thick. They have an irregular outer appearance resulting from deposition of scar tissue where follicles have previously ruptured.

The outer surface of the ovary is formed of a layer of columnar cells and is known as the germinal epithelium. This is a misnomer; it was originally thought that the ova were produced in this layer but this is not so. Next there is a poorly defined layer of fibrous connective tissue – the tunica albuginea – and then the cortex where the female germ cells (oocytes) are located and develop. The innermost layer is the vascular medulla (Fig 1.10).

A **follicle** consists of the developing oocyte and its surrounding follicular cells, and changes occur in both during the ovulatory cycle. The primordial follicle consists of flat cuboidal cells and these divide to form several layers of granulosa cells in the primary follicle. Amorphous material begins to accumulate between the granulosa cells and the oocyte, known as the **zona pellucida**. Outside the

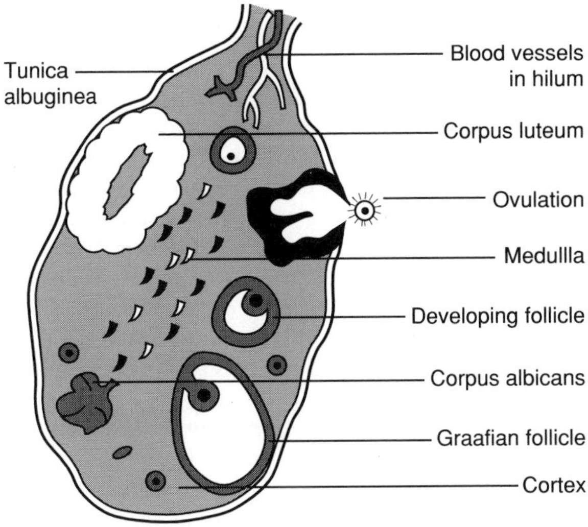

Fig. 1.10 General plan of the ovary.

follicle the interstitial cells change to become the theca folliculi which is then invaded by capillaries. The inner layer of the theca produces oestrogens. The follicle continues to increase in size and an antrum, or cleft, appears which fills with follicular fluid. At this stage the structure is known as the **secondary follicle**. After a further period of maturation the granulosa cells split: one layer forms the corona radiata around the oocyte and the other outer layer, the membrana granulosa. The two layers are continuous at the cumulus oophorus. At this stage the whole structure is called a **Graafian follicle**, which gradually moves towards the surface of the ovary.

Simultaneously, a mature **ovum** is developing within the follicle. The primordial germ cells differentiate into **oogonia** and by the third month of the intrauterine life of the fetus they begin to undergo mitotic division to form primary **oocytes**. The primary oocytes are located in the primordial follicle. The first meiotic division occurs at this stage. Meiosis in the primary oocyte begins *in utero* and division up to the diplotene stage of prophase I is completed shortly before birth. Then there is a long resting phase; in the case of the human oocyte it may be anywhere between 10 and 50 years. Thus the first meiotic division is not completed until around the time of ovulation.

In each ovarian cycle some 20 or so oocytes become selectively reactivated and proceed through meiotic division. However, usually only one continues through to the Graafian follicle stage, probably from alternate ovaries. The first meiotic division is completed before ovulation, giving a **secondary oocyte** (with only 23 chromosomes) and the **first polar body** (a polar body is a minute cell containing one of the nuclei formed during meiotic cell division, but virtually no cytoplasm; the secondary oocyte retains the major portion of cytoplasm). The second meiotic division begins almost immediately, but stops again at metaphase II and there is another, comparatively short, resting phase until fertilization. So the secondary oocyte (with the first polar body still in the zona pellucida) is released from the Graafian follicle at ovulation. Completion of the second meiotic division is dependent upon fertilization, that is, penetration of the ovum by a spermatozoon.

The exact mechanism of **ovulation** – the release of the ovum from the Graafian follicle (in fact as a secondary oocyte) – is not fully understood but it probably results from increasing quantities of follicular fluid which raise the pressure and cause the follicle to burst. Prostaglandins may well be involved in the process of follicular rupture. Other biologically active substances have also been found in follicular fluid. The hormone inhibin found first in males has been isolated in relatively high concentrations in female follicular fluid and it appears that inhibin is at least one of the factors which determines the number of follicles released at ovulation. In this way interference with the action of inhibin might contribute to the regulation of fertility (de Jong, 1987). (Inhibin may also have a role in polycystic ovarian disease.)

The follicle, a fluid-filled mass, just before rupture is approximately 2 cm in diameter – this is large enough to be picked up by ultrasound. The secondary oocyte, together with its follicular cells of the cumulus, is released into the abdominal cavity after which it is usually trapped by the fimbriae of the uterine tube. After ovulation the follicle collapses and the membrana granulosa becomes folded.

It is difficult to be certain on clinical grounds that ovulation has occurred: up to 10% of ovarian cycles can be anovulatory, that is, no follicle ruptures (Wilson & Rennie, 1976). The only absolute proof is pregnancy, but a regular cycle and dysmenorrhoea (see section on menstrual cycle) are indications that cycles are ovulatory. Some women notice lower abdominal pain for a brief period at ovulation, known as **mittelschmerz** (German for middle pain). The pain may be bilateral or unilateral. It is usually cramp-like and lasts a day or so and is often replaced by a dull ache. The cause of the pain is uncertain: it may be due to some local irritation within the pelvis caused by the presence of follicular fluid and blood, or from the ovary itself. Most women have some microscopic bleeding into the vagina at that time and a few experience overt bleeding; this is probably due to a temporary fall in sex hormone production between the time of the follicle rupturing and before the establishment of a corpus luteum (Fig. 1.11).

The collapsed follicle becomes an endocrine gland and is termed the **corpus luteum** or yellow body (the yellowish carotenoid pigment, lutein, is formed within the cells). Both the granulosa and theca cells proliferate. The corpus luteum secretes the steroids oestrogen and progesterone and both play an important role in the reproductive cycle and in the maintenance of pregnancy should fertilization occur (androgens are also secreted from the stroma of the ovary). The corpus luteum, however, has a finite life, the length of which depends on whether pregnancy occurs or not. If no pregnancy ensues, the lutein cells degenerate after approximately 12–14 days and hormone production is reduced. Accompanying this degeneration, the corpus luteum becomes infiltrated by fibroblasts that produce scar tissue and it becomes known as the **corpus albicans** (the white body). If pregnancy occurs, the corpus luteum persists and continues to secrete oestrogen and progesterone until about the third month of gestation, when the fetoplacental unit assumes this function (see later).

The cycle of events previously described is known as the **ovarian** or **ovulatory**

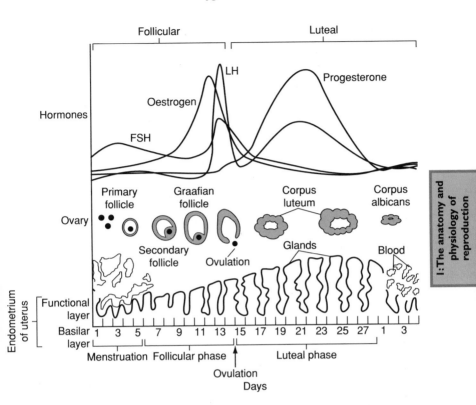

Fig. 1.11 The menstrual cycle showing the precisely synchronized events that take place within the pituitary, ovary and uterus. The cycle repeats about every 28 days if fertilization does not take place.

cycle. The cycle lasts approximately 28 days in most women, although it can vary between 21 and 35 days. It is usually divided into two phases.

The **follicular phase**, when the ovarian follicles grow, mature and finally rupture; during this time the theca interna cells secrete oestrogen.

The **luteal phase**, when the formation, development and degeneration of the corpus luteum occur; the granulosa lutein cells secrete progesterone and the theca lutein cells secrete oestrogens (Fig. 1.11).

The luteal phase of the cycle lasts approximately 14 days, although slight variations do occur amongst different individuals and from cycle to cycle in one individual; the follicular phase is more variable and accounts for the wide range in cycle length. To determine the timing of ovulation it is usual to count *back* 14 days from the first day of the next menstruation.

Successful release of a secondary oocyte from a mature Graafian follicle is dependent upon the appropriate level of circulating gonadotrophins from the anterior pituitary and this is first achieved around the time of puberty (during the years from birth until puberty some follicular growth and activity occur in the ovary but follicles degenerate before completing their development).

The gonadotrophins involved are **follicle-stimulating hormone** (FSH) and **luteinizing hormone** (LH). FSH stimulates the initial development of the follicles, but the process is *not* completed to the Graafian follicle stage. Subsequent release of FSH leads to completion of follicular growth, ovulation, and development of a corpus luteum. LH then maintains the corpus luteum, stimulating the release of progesterone and oestrogens. It is now generally accepted that it is a surge in the level of LH that causes ovulation. There is a smaller peak in FSH release but this is probably due to the secretion of only one releasing hormone from the hypothalamus that raises both LH and FSH levels at the same time (see Fig. 1.11). (A fuller description of the hormonal control is given after discussion of the menstrual cycle.) Ovulation predictor kits are available over the counter at chemists for women to use at home; they work by measuring levels of LH. The test detects the sudden surge or increase of LH around the middle of the cycle; ovulation occurs 24–36 hours after the surge and this is the time of peak fertility.

The menstrual cycle

The hormones released by the ovaries have functional and structural repercussions throughout the body, but particularly on the reproductive system. The changes occurring in the endometrium of the uterus constitute the menstrual cycle, which terminates in the loss of blood per vagina, i.e. menstruation. The length of the cycle is said to be approximately 28 days but its actual length may vary considerably, and 24–32 days is quite normal.

The menstrual cycle is usually divided into three phases: the proliferative, secretory and menstrual phases (see Fig. 1.11). The **proliferative phase**, which lasts 10–11 days, coincides with the growth of the ovarian follicles and the secretion of oestrogenic hormones. The endometrium is gradually built up from the stratum basale, the epithelium regenerates from the stumps of the uterine glands left from the previous cycle, and the vascularity of the stroma increases. All these changes are brought about by the influence of oestrogens. By the time the Graafian follicle is fully mature, the regenerative changes in the uterus are complete.

The next stage is the **secretory phase** and it coincides with the period when the corpus luteum is functionally active and secreting progesterone and oestrogens and lasts for approximately 14 days. Under the influence of these hormones, particularly progesterone, the cells of the endometrial stroma become oedematous, the glands dilate and secrete a glycogen-rich watery mucus and the spiral arteries become increasingly prominent and tightly coiled. These spiral arteries undergo rhythmic dilations and contractions which are under the control of the ovarian hormones. The endometrium is approximately 5 mm thick at this stage.

After approximately 12–14 days, if fertilization has not occurred, the corpus luteum begins to degenerate and the secretion of ovarian hormones wanes. Thus the hormonal support of the endometrial tissue is withdrawn; there is a loss of water and a decreased blood flow to the endometrium due to spasm of the spiral arteries, which ultimately leads to endometrial necrosis (death of the tissue). However, when the endometrial arteries dilate again bleeding occurs into the stroma of the necrotic endometrium. Thus blood enters the lumen of the uterus and menstruation, or the menstrual phase, commences. The endometrium produces prostaglandins in increasing amounts during the secretory phase and these reach a peak at the time of menstruation. It is possible that prostaglandins are involved in the initiation of menstruation and the shedding of the endometrium.

Other changes associated with the ovarian and menstrual cycles

Changes occur in other regions of the reproductive system, also under the influence of the ovarian hormones. During the follicular phase the epithelium of the uterine tubes proliferates and during the luteal phase the secretory cells become more active, presumably to supply nutrients for the ovum as it moves to the uterus. There are changes in the motility of the muscular elements of the uterine tubes and uterus: tubal movements and myometrial contractions predominate under oestrogenic influence, whilst progesterone decreases the motility. Again it has been suggested that prostaglandins may be involved in tubal contractility and ovum transport.

Cyclical changes are seen in the composition of the mucus secreted by the cervix (the cervix itself does not exhibit marked cyclical activity). As a result of the oestrogen secretion at the time of ovulation, the water and electrolyte content of the mucus increases. This thinner mucus, produced around the time of ovulation, is thought to allow easier penetration of the cervix by spermatozoa. During the luteal phase, under the influence of progesterone, the volume of mucus decreases and it becomes thicker. At the time of ovulation, the mucus develops the property of 'spinnbarkheit', which means that it can be drawn out into long threads.

There are marked changes in the squamous epithelial cells of the vagina during the menstrual cycle. Under oestrogenic stimulation, there is an increased tendency to cornification (an increase in 'horny' tissue) of the cells which decreases under the influence of progesterone. This change may increase the vagina's resistance to trauma.

The breasts may increase in size and tenderness in the premenstrual week, due to oedema and hyperaemia (increased blood flow) in the intralobular connective tissue. There is often an increase in skin pigmentation pre-menstrually, especially around the eyes, but also in the areola of the nipple. These changes may be due to an increase in the level of melanocyte-stimulating hormone from the anterior pituitary, and are similar to those seen in pregnancy, but less marked.

The integration of the hormonal systems

Several components of the hormonal systems involved in female reproductive physiology have been discussed in isolation, but it is crucial to understand the integration and interrelationships of these systems (see Table 1.1). Gonadotrophins from the anterior pituitary induce both ovulation and the secretion of the ovarian hormones, and these in turn have widespread effects on the body. But how are all these events coordinated?

The hypothalamus is the vital integrating centre. The release of gonadotrophins FSH and LH from the pituitary is controlled by a releasing hormone produced in the median eminence of the hypothalamus. There appears to be

1: The anatomy and physiology of reproduction

Table 1.1 Principal female reproductive hormones

Endocrine gland and hormone	Principal target tissue	Principal actions
Hypothalamus		
Gonadotrophin releasing hormone (GnRH)	Anterior pituitary	Stimulates release of FSH and LH
Anterior pituitary		
Follicle-stimulating hormone (FSH)	Ovary	Stimulates development of follicles; with LH, stimulates secretion of oestrogens and ovulation
Luteinizing hormone (LH)	Ovary	Stimulates final development of follicle; stimulates ovulation; stimulates development of corpus luteum
Prolactin	Breasts	Stimulates milk production (after breast has been prepared by oestrogens and progesterone)
Posterior pituitary		
Oxytocin	Breasts	Stimulates release of milk into ducts
	Uterus	Stimulates contraction
Ovary		
Oestrogens	General	Growth of body and sex organs at puberty; development of secondary sex characteristics (breast development, broadening pelvis, distribution of fat and muscle)
	Reproductive structures	Maturation; monthly preparation of the endometrium for pregnancy; makes cervical mucus thinner and more alkaline
Progesterone	Uterus	Completes preparation of and maintains endometrium for pregnancy
	Breasts	Stimulates development of lobules and alveoli of mammary glands

only one hormone produced and this one hormone stimulates the release of both FSH and LH at the same time. Hence it is given the name gonadotrophin-releasing hormone (GnRH) or sometimes follicle-stimulating hormone/luteinizing hormone-releasing hormone (FSH/LH-RH).

The release of GnRH from the hypothalamus causes the release of FSH and LH from the anterior pituitary, which in turn causes development of the ovarian follicles, release of an ovum, maintenance of the corpus luteum and, as a result, the secretion of oestrogens and progesterone. The regulation and integration of this system are complicated, involving fine balances between the levels of gonadotrophins and ovarian hormones, incorporating both negative and positive feedback pathways and influences from other parts of the brain. The important sensor in the system is the part of the hypothalamus that is sensitive to circulating levels of oestrogens. It is logical for oestrogen to be the important factor, as oestrogen levels give a direct indication of the stage of follicular development and are also responsible for producing most of the preparatory changes necessary to ensure fertilization.

When there are low levels of circulating oestrogens, during and following menstruation, a negative feedback system operates, i.e. the hypothalamus detects the low oestrogen levels and release of GnRH is increased. This is turn increases secretion of FSH, which stimulates follicular development (in the presence of basal levels of LH). Several follicles begin to develop during each cycle under the influence of FSH and they all contribute initially to the increasing oestrogen levels. The higher level of oestrogen is then detected by the hypothalamus and levels of FSH are subsequently reduced; only the most mature follicle will be able to complete its development without the FSH stimulus; the other follicles degenerate (Fig. 1.12).

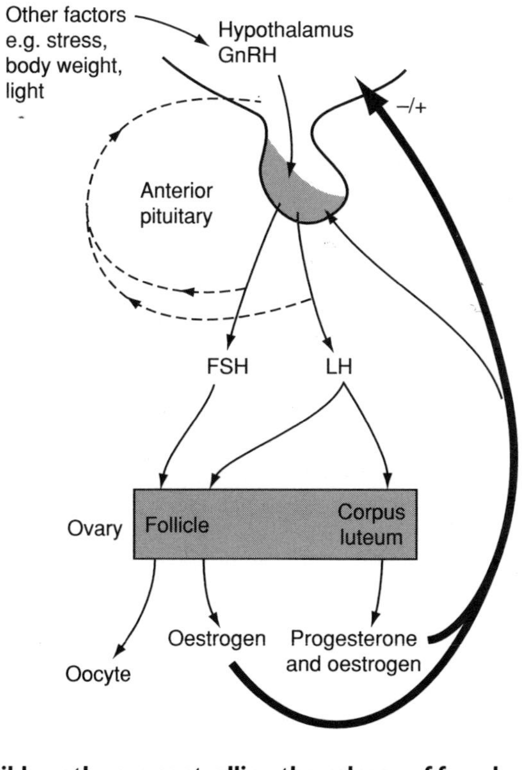

Fig. 1.12 Possible pathways controlling the release of female reproductive hormones. GnRH = gonadotrophin-releasing hormone; FSH = follicle-stimulating hormone; LH = luteinizing hormone.

Oestrogen probably affects both the anterior pituitary and the hypothalamus, although the latter is thought to be the main site of action. There may also be a short feedback loop, with levels of LH and FSH directly influencing release of GnRH.

However, a simple negative feedback loop is not an adequate explanation. The LH surge that produces ovulation (see Fig. 1.11) is due to a positive feedback mechanism, that is, *high* oestrogen levels, acting on the hypothalamus, produce the surge in LH secretion (the second surge of FSH is presumably a result of the surge in releasing hormone and is of secondary importance to the LH surge). The precise mechanism for this paradoxical negative/positive feedback system is uncertain and many aspects require confirmation by further research. The proposed mechanism stated here is no doubt a gross simplification of the complex monitoring system involved.

External stimuli are also known to affect the occurrence and timing of ovulation and menstruation. Ovulation is commonly delayed in females subject to mild stress, for example when taking examinations, and it may cease altogether under conditions of severe stress, for example some women in prisoner-of-war camps ceased to menstruate.

The female reproductive system is thus governed by a complex control system, the main points of which can be summarized as follows (Fig. 1.13).

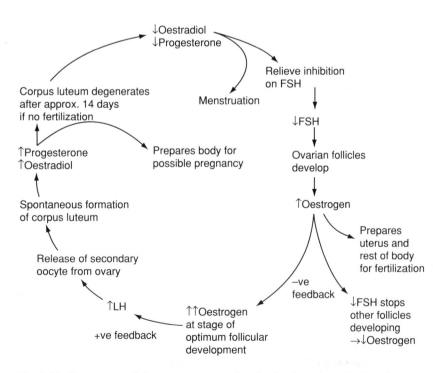

Fig. 1.13 Summary of the events occurring in the female reproductive system.

1. Falling oestrogen and progesterone levels initiate menstruation and also relieve the inhibition on FSH secretion; thus FSH levels rise and follicles begin to develop.

2. As the follicles mature, increasing levels of oestrogen are secreted which in turn inhibits the secretion of FSH (the negative feedback in operation); oestrogen also prepares the uterus and the rest of the body for ovulation.

3. As a result of optimum follicular maturation, oestrogen levels rise high enough at mid cycle to stimulate the release of sufficient LH to result in ovulation. This forms the positive feedback mechanism of oestrogen on the hypothalamus.

4. A corpus luteum forms spontaneously from the collapsed follicle after ovulation and secretes progesterone and oestrogen, which maintain the suppression of the gonadotrophins and prepare the body for possible pregnancy.

5. In the absence of fertilization and the implantation of the embryo, the corpus luteum degenerates and the levels of ovarian hormones fall, inducing endometrial breakdown.

6. The cycle is repeated.

The menopause

The menopause is a single event occurring during the **climacteric**, a period which extends for some years either side of the menopause. The menopause is the permanent cessation of menstruation resulting from loss of ovarian activity. By definition, it must be a retrospective diagnosis because 12 months of amenorrhoea must follow the last menses in order to assume safely that periods have ceased (WHO, 1981). The systemic changes associated with it may occur months before or after the cessation of menstruation; therefore the term menopause is often used to embrace both the last menses and the changes that occur. It can take 5–7 years for all the changes to be complete.

During the climacteric, ovulation ceases and there is a deficiency of oestrogen and progesterone. The hypothalamus and anterior pituitary respond to this deficiency by increasing secretions of GnRH, and FSH and LH, respectively. This increased output of gonadotrophins, which can reach ten times the level in a normal menstruating woman, remains raised for some 20 years or so until senescence occurs. The menopausal symptoms are caused by the deficiency of ovarian hormones and the increase in FSH and LH. For reasons not yet understood, the ovary becomes resistant to stimuli from the pituitary gland and oestrogen levels fall. In its efforts to stimulate the ovary to work, increased levels of human menopausal gonadotrophin (hMG) are produced by the pituitary gland (McEwan, 1990). FSH and hMG are very similar. The decline in oestrogen is normally gradual, although it is rapid where a pre-menopausal woman has her ovaries removed surgically. Oestrogen is still produced after the menopause, not in the ovaries but in glands such as the adrenal gland and also in adipose tissue.

The human is probably the only animal which has a significant period of life beyond the cessation of reproductive ability. In the majority of women, the

1:The anatomy and physiology of reproduction

menopause occurs between the ages of 45 and 55 years, but it can occur anywhere between 40 and 55 years. In the UK, the mean age of menopause is around 48 years (Dalton, 1983). Pregnancy resulting in a spontaneous abortion has been reliably reported as late as the age of 56 years.

THE PHYSIOLOGY OF SEXUAL INTERCOURSE

The male and female gametes are brought together by the act of sexual intercourse (**coitus**). A brief description of the events of coitus will now be given.

The male

1:The anatomy and physiology of reproduction

The normal state of the penis is flaccid, but under conditions of sexual excitement it becomes erect. **Erection** is purely a vascular phenomenon: during sexual excitement, the arterioles in the erectile tissue of the penis (corpus spongiosum and corpora cavernosa, see Fig. 1.4) dilate and become engorged with blood. As the erectile bodies are surrounded by a strong fibrous coat the penis becomes rigid, elongated and increases in girth. As the erectile tissue expands, the veins emptying the corpora are compressed and thus the outflow of blood is minimal. The process occurs rapidly, in 5–10 seconds. Erection is controlled by a spinal reflex.

The erection reflex (Fig. 1.14) can start from direct stimulation of the genitals – the glans penis or the skin around the genitals. There are highly sensitive mechanoreceptors located in the tip of the penis. The afferent synapse in the lower spinal cord and the efferent flow, via the nervi erigentes, produce relaxation of the arterioles in the penis. The higher brain centres, via descending pathways, can have profound facilitative or inhibitory effects. Thoughts, visual cues or emotions can cause erection in the complete absence of any mechanical stimulation.

The parasympathetic nerves simultaneously stimulate the urethral glands to secrete a mucoid-like material which aids lubrication. Erection allows entry of

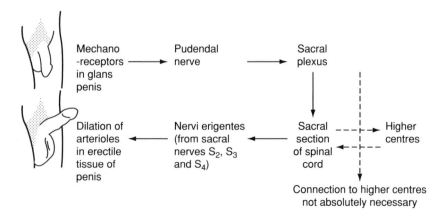

Fig. 1.14 The nervous pathways (simplified) involved in the erection reflex.

the penis into the female vagina, and the angle which the erect penis makes with the male's trunk closely follows the angle of the vagina in the female's pelvis.

After intromission (the insertion of the erect penis into the vagina), **ejaculation of semen** into the female vagina may occur. This is again basically a spinal reflex and the afferent pathway is the same as for erection. When the level of stimulation reaches a critical peak, a patterned automatic sequence of efferent discharge is elicited to the smooth muscle of the genital ducts and to the skeletal muscle at the base of the penis. The exact nature of the nervous pathways involved is complex but includes sympathetic stimulation to the ducts, via L_1 and L_2 nerve roots. The first stage is known as emission, and the genital ducts and accessory glands empty their contents into the posterior urethra. During the second stage, ejaculation proper, the semen is expelled from the penis, by a series of rapid muscle contractions, into the female genital tract.

During ejaculation the sphincter at the base of the bladder is closed, therefore no spermatozoa can enter the bladder nor can urine be voided. This again is under the control of the sympathetic nervous system. A feeling of intense pleasure arises with ejaculation and the event is referred to as an **orgasm**. There is simultaneously a noticeable skeletal muscle contraction throughout the body which is rapidly followed by muscular and psychological relaxation. After ejaculation there is a **latent period** during which time a second erection is not possible. The latent period varies from individual to individual but can range from a few minutes to several hours in 'normal' men. Loss of erection occurs due to vasoconstriction of the arterioles in the penis, hence venous compression is reduced.

Any interference with the spinal reflexes may result in impotence or other sexual dysfunction (although libido is unaffected). For example, ejaculation is usually not possible after a bilateral lumbar sympathectomy below L_2. Erection may not be possible after an abdominoperineal resection due to damage to the nervi erigentes. Administration of drugs that inhibit the release of noradrenaline from postganglionic sympathetic nerve endings, e.g. methyldopa and reserpine, can lead to ejaculatory failure, although erection and sensation would be normal. Ganglion-blocking drugs, e.g. hexamethonium, inhibit both parasympathetic and sympathetic nerve pathways and reduce both erection and ejaculation; these drugs are rarely used now because of their widespread anticholinergic side effects.

It is worth noting that hypertensive individuals report few problems in sexual performance whilst undiagnosed, and thus untreated, but once hypotensive therapy has been initiated, the incidence of impotence and erection failure increases considerably due to the nature of the drugs prescribed. Diabetic patients also suffer from problems with impotence, although the cause is probably a result of metabolic, neuropathological and vascular disturbance. Some patients who have spinal cord injuries have problems too. The extent of return to normal sexual function in these patients varies considerably according to the nature and position of the injury: Trimmer (1978) estimates that erections return eventually in approximately 75% of cases, but there is a low incidence of orgasm. Sex education and counselling for patients with all types of handicap are important. There are several organizations that can help patients.

The female

In the female, sexual excitement is characterized by erection of the clitoris and labia minora, both of which are largely composed of erectile tissue. The neural control of erection is the same as for the male. The breasts may enlarge during sexual excitement and the nipples become erect. As the sexual tension increases, there may be a flushing of the skin which begins on the chest and spreads upwards over the breasts, neck and up to the face.

The female provides most of the lubrication for coitus by the transudation of fluid through the vaginal walls. The exact source of the mucus is unclear as there are no glands in the vagina. Additional secretions may come from the glands in the vulva and from the Bartholin's glands.

The movement of the penis in and out of the vagina causes pleasure in both the male and female. The female may experience a climax (or orgasm) similar to that of the male. Stimulation of the clitoris may heighten the state of excitement and contributes to the orgasm of the female. The female is potentially capable of several orgasms within a short period of time, unlike the male. During coitus and orgasm the uterus may contract rhythmically and this may serve to aspirate the semen into the uterine lumen. Females do not always experience orgasm, and it is not necessary for successful fertilization; for example, orgasm does not occur in artificial insemination. Orgasm may, however, contribute to fertilization in some cases of subfertility where uterine aspirations hasten the movement of spermatozoa towards the ovum.

CONCEPTION

The egg is released from the ovary at the second metaphase stage of meiosis and it enters the uterine tube still surrounded by follicular cells. If **fertilization** occurs, it does so in the ampulla of the uterine tube.

Normally the spermatozoa reach the oocyte by traversing the lumen of the uterus and moving along the uterine tubes. Estimates vary, but spermatozoa on their own can probably move only a few millimetres per hour, by propelled movement of their tails. The fact that after coitus spermatozoa can reach the ampulla of the uterine tube within 30 minutes or so implies that their movement is assisted. As already discussed, coitus provides the initial impetus to spermatozoa in their journey. After coitus, the primary transport mechanism is contraction of the musculature in the uterus and uterine tubes. Prostaglandins present in the semen may cause the smooth muscle to contract. The wastage rate of spermatozoa is huge: of the several hundred million spermatozoa deposited in the vagina, only a few thousand actually reach the uterine tubes.

As the spermatozoa are transported to the site of fertilization, they undergo their final maturation which enables them to pass through the follicular cells and zona pellucida and penetrate the oocyte. The maturation processes are known as **capacitation** and the **acrosome reaction**. These processes involve changes in the acrosome and the release of hyaluronidase and other proteolytic enzymes which assist the passage of the spermatozoa through the layers of cells around the oocyte. It has been postulated that a high density of spermatozoa is required to produce sufficient hyaluronidase to remove most of the follicular cells. However, only one spermatozoon is able to enter one egg. The entry of additional spermatozoa appears to be blocked in some way.

The time available for fertilization of the oocyte in the female is approximately 24 hours after ovulation, after which time the egg begins to degenerate. Spermatozoa maintain their fertilizing ability for up to 48 hours (some suggest even as long as 72 hours) inside the female genital tract, so there is only a limited period when fertilization is at all possible.

The penetration of the oocyte by the head of the spermatozoon is followed by completion of the second meiotic division of the ovum and the formation of the second polar body. The nuclei of the spermatozoon and ovum, containing the maternal and paternal haploid sets of chromosomes, come together on the mitotic spindle. Fertilization is completed with the restoration of the diploid complement of chromosomes.

The role of the uterine or Fallopian tubes is much more than that of a simple muscular tube – they play an important part not only in ensuring fertilization occurs, but also in the first few days after fertilization. For example, appropriate muscular contraction and ciliary movement are necessary and there needs to be the correct volume and concentration of fluid in the tubes; this fluid probably has some nutritional role and may also convey biochemical signals which condition subsequent events such as capacitation and cleavage in the gametes. It is thought that tubal activities are probably controlled by the ovary.

HORMONE CHANGES DURING PREGNANCY

The hormone changes during pregnancy are many and complex, and much still remains to be learned about them. Progesterone and oestrogen are essential for the initiation and continuance of pregnancy. Fertilization results in the persistence of the corpus luteum which continues to develop and increases its secretion of these hormones. Progesterone maintains the endometrium in its 'progestational' state essential for pregnancy, and is necessary to depress the contractile activity of the uterus, thus allowing the blastocyst to implant and preventing its expulsion. Oestrogens are necessary for uterine growth, which involves both general protein synthesis and the production of specific enzymes necessary for muscular contraction and energy mechanisms – these are important during parturition. The arbortifacient known as Mifegyne is a synthetic antiprogesterone drug; if Mifegyne is administered in early pregnancy it blocks the action of progesterone and results in abortion. This demonstrates that progesterone is vital in early pregnancy.

The non-pregnant corpus luteum is maintained by the gonadotrophin LH from the anterior pituitary. However, LH levels fall 12–14 days after ovulation. The corpus luteum is maintained in a pregnant woman by **human chorionic gonadotrophin** (hCG), produced by the trophoblast of the developing blastocyst. hCG is a glycoprotein very similar in structure to LH and is found only in the presence of a trophoblast. It can be detected in maternal blood and urine about 10 days after ovulation, i.e. 5 days before the next menstrual period would have occurred. Thus the blastocyst must begin to produce hCG very soon after fertilization and before implantation is complete. hCG maintains the secretion of progesterone and oestrogen from the corpus luteum in early pregnancy.

Secretion of hCG reaches a peak 8–9 weeks after the last menstrual period and then the level drops dramatically to a lower one that is maintained until the end of pregnancy (Fig. 1.15). Thus the function of the corpus luteum also begins to decline after 8 weeks of pregnancy. Oophorectomy (excision of an ovary) before the sixth week leads to abortion, but after that time has no effect on pregnancy.

In humans the placenta takes over steroid production from the corpus luteum by the twelfth week of pregnancy. Oestrogen, particularly oestriol, and progesterone are synthesized in the placenta from precursors originating mainly from the fetal adrenal glands and liver and from the maternal adrenal glands. It is likely that the placental hormones are synthesized and released by the syncytiotrophoblast, the outer layer of the trophoblast. The interdependence of fetal and placental tissues for the production of oestrogen in particular has given rise to the concept of the **fetoplacental unit**, the term implying that both are necessary and neither can function in isolation.

Progesterone and oestrogen levels rise throughout pregnancy until just prior to delivery and these elevated levels inhibit the release of FSH and LH.

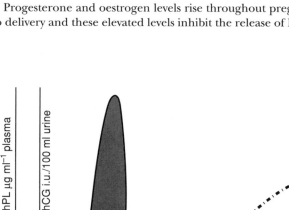

Fig. 1.15 Changes in hormone levels during pregnancy. hCG = human chorionic gonadotrophin; hPL = human placental lactogen.

Another hormone produced by the fetoplacental unit is **human placental lactogen** (hPL), also known as human chorionic somatomammotrophin (hCS). Levels of hPL rise steadily throughout pregnancy, with the curve flattening off towards term (see Fig. 1.15). hPL is structurally very similar to growth hormone. The exact role of hPL is unknown but it exhibits growth-promoting and lactogenic (able to induce lactation) properties.

Maternal oxytocin levels rise throughout pregnancy. **Oxytocin**, secreted from the posterior pituitary gland, stimulates the contraction of the smooth muscle of the pregnant uterus and lactating mammary glands, but this effect is held in check by the high levels of progesterone that inhibit uterine motility. Only at parturition is oxytocin left unopposed to act on the smooth muscle of the uterus.

ACKNOWLEDGEMENTS

This chapter has been adapted from *Physiology for Nursing Practice*, 2nd edition, edited by Susan M. Hinchcliff, Susan E. Montague and Roger Watson (Baillière Tindall, London, 1996).

1: The anatomy and physiology of reproduction

NATURAL FAMILY PLANNING METHODS: FERTILITY AWARENESS

2

INTRODUCTION

Natural family planning methods have been used widely in the past by various religious groups such as the Roman Catholic faith. They involve the observation of certain body changes which denote ovulation. From this information a couple may choose to either abstain from sexual intercourse and use it as their family planning method, or use this fertile period to have sexual intercourse promoting pregnancy, known as fertility awareness.

HISTORY

Natural family planning methods have been referred to previously as periodic abstinence, the safe period and the rhythm method. It is only more recently that it has been promoted to women as a fertility awareness method, and as more women are delaying pregnancy this has become a popular choice. Infertility clinics may ask women at initial consultations to use fertility awareness kits; previously they used the temperature method to indicate ovulation.

In 1930 Ogino in Japan and in 1933 Knaus in Austria found that conception took place in-between menstrual cycles, and the time from ovulation to the next menstrual period was always the same regardless of the cycle. Using this information they developed the calendar method. Around this period changes in the cervical mucus were noted by Seguy and Vimeux. Ferin in 1947 first noticed that a woman's body temperature changed at ovulation. However, it was not until 1964 that Drs John and Evelyn Billings used these discoveries to formulate the Billings method, now known as the cervical method.

Recently research has increased in this area producing personal contraceptive systems and urinary dipsticks. The temperature method has benefited from electronic and digital thermometers by increasing accuracy and decreasing the time clients need to take their temperature.

EXPLANATION OF THE METHOD

There are four main natural family planning and fertility awareness methods:

1. The temperature method
2. The cervical mucus method (previously known as the Billings method)
3. The calendar method
4. Combination of methods, also known as the sympto-thermal method or double-check method.

These methods help a woman to recognize when ovulation takes place. This usually occurs between days 12 and 16 before the next menstrual period. The ovum remains capable of being fertilized for 12–24 hours, whilst sperm are capable of fertilizing the ovum for 3–5 days and on occasions have survived up to 7 days *in utero* (see Fig. 2.1).

During each menstrual cycle the pituitary gland releases **follicle-stimulating hormone** (FSH). This triggers the development of follicles which contain the immature ova and is known as the **follicular phase**. As the follicles develop they secrete the hormone oestrogen. This causes the reduction of FSH so that further ovum development is inhibited, the endometrium becomes thickened ready for implantation, and the cervical glands produce mucus favourable to sperm penetration. As the ovum ripens the level of oestrogen rises, causing the pituitary gland to produce **luteinizing hormone (LH)**. This causes the follicle to rupture, releasing the ovum into the fallopian tube; this is known as **ovulation**. Rising oestrogen levels cause the cervix to soften and rise upwards and the **os** to open. The empty follicle becomes the **corpus luteum**, which secretes the hormone progesterone. This part of the menstrual cycle is known as the **luteal phase**. Progesterone causes the basal body temperature to rise during the luteal phase after ovulation. The

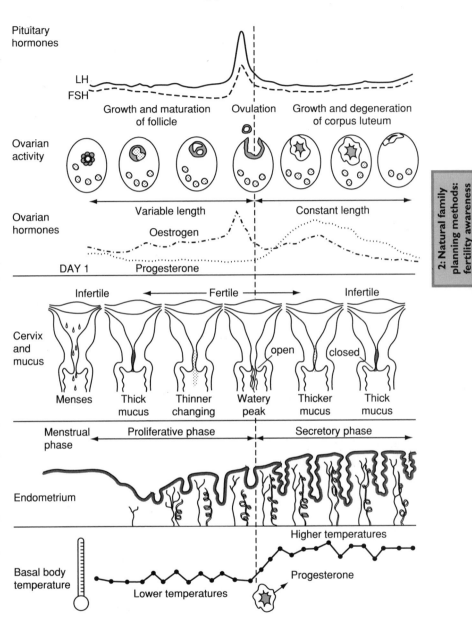

Fig. 2.1 Changes during the menstrual cycle. (Reproduced with kind permission from 'Fertility' – Fertility Awareness and Natural Family Planning 3rd edition, Dr E. Clubb & J. Knight, 1996, David & Charles.)

2: Natural family planning methods: fertility awareness

pituitary gland is now inhibited from producing LH and FSH so that further ovulation is prevented. Following ovulation cervical mucus becomes thickened and sticky, making sperm penetration difficult. The cervix becomes firm and the os closes. If the ovum is fertilized then the corpus luteum will continue to produce progesterone throughout early pregnancy. However if the ovum is not fertilized then the corpus luteum will disintegrate, the level of progesterone will drop and menstruation will occur. The shift in basal body temperature, position of the cervix and change in cervical mucus are all used as indicators for natural family planning and fertility awareness to assess when a woman is fertile.

EFFICACY

The efficacy of natural family planning methods is 80–98% with careful use. The sympto-thermal is the most effective method as it uses a combination of methods. In theory the efficacy of the sympto-thermal method can be as high as 98%; however, with this and any natural family planning method the range of effectiveness of the method is dependent on the user, and is known as the user failure rate. The efficacy is dependent on the level of motivation and commitment the couple give to the method. Many men and women use this method to space their pregnancies, and as a result may be prepared to take more risks – a pregnancy slightly earlier than planned may be a happy accident! However, couples who are using the method to avoid pregnancy are more likely to be highly motivated and conscientious; they are less likely to take risks so the user failure rate will be lower and the efficacy higher. Lastly the level and expertise of the teaching of this method will influence the efficacy of the method, which is why it is vital that this method is taught by a teacher trained in natural family planning.

DISADVANTAGES OF NATURAL FAMILY PLANNING METHODS

❖ Requires motivation
❖ Needs to be taught by a specialist in natural family planning
❖ Requires the observation and recording of changes in the body
❖ May take time to learn so may require a period of abstinence.

ADVANTAGES OF NATURAL FAMILY PLANNING METHODS

❖ Once learnt it is under the control of the couple
❖ Inexpensive (except in the personal contraceptive method)
❖ Can be used to promote pregnancy
❖ Increases couple's knowledge of changes in the body and fertility
❖ No physical side effects
❖ Acceptable to some religious beliefs and cultures

THE TEMPERATURE METHOD

The temperature method involves the woman taking her temperature every day to record her basal body temperature. Following ovulation the basal body temperature (BBT) will drop slightly and then rise by 0.2–0.4°C where it will stay until the next period. This occurs because after ovulation the hormone progesterone is secreted by the corpus luteum which causes a woman's basal body temperature to rise (see Fig. 2.1).

The client should be advised to take her temperature at the same time each day before getting out of bed. If she works night shift she should do this after sleeping in the evening. She should take her temperature first before drinking or eating as these will affect the basal body temperature. The thermometer should be an ovulation thermometer which is calibrated in tenths of a degree between the range of 35 and 39°C. A digital or electronic thermometer may be used which takes about 45 seconds to give a reading. The temperature can be taken orally which takes 5 minutes, or vaginally or rectally which takes 3 minutes. The temperature should always be taken by the same route to avoid inaccuracy. The temperature is recorded on a chart commencing on the first day of her menstrual period (see Fig. 2.2). Once the temperature has risen and has been maintained for 3 days then the couple may have unprotected sexual intercourse until the first day of the next menstrual period.

Disadvantages

❖ Requires motivation

❖ Needs to be taught by a specialist in natural family planning

❖ The basal body temperature is affected by illness, disturbed sleep, stress, alcohol and drugs e.g. aspirin

❖ If the temperature is not taken at roughly the same time each day this will lead to inaccuracies in the BBT

❖ Does not detect the beginning of the fertile period, making it harder to achieve pregnancy

❖ Requires long periods of abstinence, as only detects post ovulation.

Advantages

❖ Increases the couple's knowledge and awareness of the fertile period

❖ Helpful to women who experience erratic cycles by detecting ovulation

❖ Can help to pinpoint other body changes such as cervical mucus

❖ Under the woman's control

❖ Can be used to prevent or promote pregnancy

CERVICAL MUCUS METHOD

The cervical mucus method involves a woman observing her cervical mucus every day. The mucus varies throughout the cycle. Following menstruation there is little

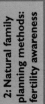

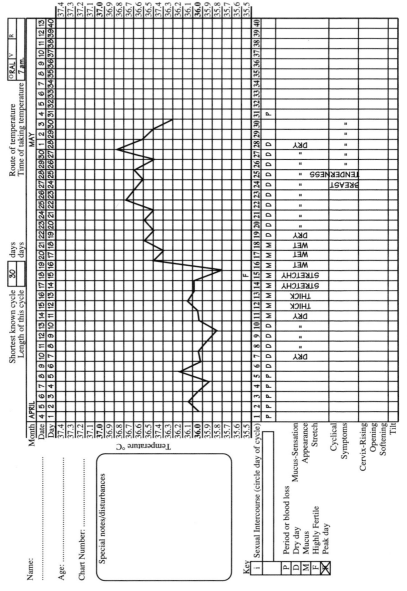

Fig. 2.2 Temperature chart.

cervical mucus and this is often described as 'dry'. The level of the hormones oestrogen and progesterone are low and the mucus is known as infertile mucus. There may be an absence of cervical mucus or it may appear sticky and if stretched between two fingers will break. As the ovum begins to ripen increasing amounts of oestrogen are produced causing an increase in cervical mucus. This marks the beginning of the fertile phase. Oestrogen levels continue to rise prior to ovulation and the cervical mucus increases in amount, becoming clear and stretchy; if held between two fingers it can stretch easily without breaking. It has been described as looking like raw egg white and is called fertile mucus. The last day of this type of mucus is known as peak mucus day; which can only be identified retrospectively. Four days following peak mucus day the mucus becomes thick, sticky and opaque and is known as infertile mucus. This change in the mucus occurs because the ovum has been released and the level of oestrogen has dropped (see Fig. 2.3).

The woman is taught to observe and record her cervical mucus several times a day either by collecting some on toilet paper or by inserting her fingers into her vagina to check its consistency and appearance. She will also be encouraged to become aware of changes in sensation of her cervical mucus. Recent trials

2: Natural family planning methods: fertility awareness

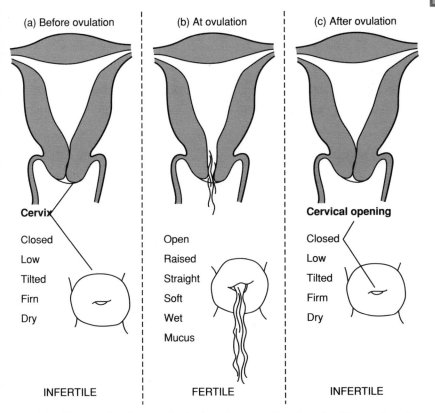

Fig. 2.3 Changes in the cervix during the menstrual cycle. (Reproduced with kind permission from 'Fertility' – Fertility Awareness and Natural Family Planning 3rd edition, Dr E. Clubb & J. Knight, 1996, David & Charles.)

(Indian Council of Medical Research Task Force on Natural Family Planning, 1996) looking at the cervical mucus method have shown a method failure rate of 1.5 per 100 users and a user failure rate of the method of 15.9 per 100 users at 21 months. This would seem to illustrate how vital training and motivation of the client and her partner are in ensuring efficacy.

Disadvantages

❖ Requires commitment
❖ Needs to be taught by a specialist in natural family planning
❖ Can take 2–3 cycles to learn method
❖ Vaginal infections can make it difficult to identify fertile mucus
❖ Some drugs used for treatment of colds etc. can inhibit cervical mucus production
❖ Involves touching the body which some women may dislike
❖ Requires abstinence.

Advantages

❖ Under the control of the woman
❖ Gives the couple permission to touch their bodies
❖ Increases awareness of body changes
❖ Predicts fertile mucus thus enabling pregnancy
❖ Can be used to prevent pregnancy.

CALENDAR METHOD

The calendar method involves a woman detecting when her fertile period is, which is usually 12–16 days before the first day of her next menstrual period. This is based on looking retrospectively over the woman's menstrual cycle for a period of 6–12 months of recorded cycles. This method is no longer recognized as reliable on its own, but may be taught alongside another method as in the combination of methods.

Disadvantages

❖ Unreliable as it does not take into account irregular cycles
❖ Stress, illness and travelling can affect the menstrual cycle
❖ Requires motivation
❖ Requires menstrual cycle to be recorded for 6–12 months prior to use.

Advantages

❖ Under the control of the woman
❖ Increases knowledge about fertility
❖ Can be used in conjunction with another method.

COMBINATION OF METHODS

This is often referred to as the sympto-thermal method or double-check method and combines the temperature, calendar and cervical mucus methods, which is why it is more effective as a contraceptive. Women are also encouraged to observe changes in their cervix such as consistency, position, and whether their cervical os is open or closed. During the beginning of the cycle when the levels of oestrogen and progesterone are reduced, the cervix is positioned low in the vagina and can be easily felt. The cervical os is closed, and the cervix feels firm to the touch. As oestrogen levels increase the cervix changes and at peak mucus day feels soft. The os is now open and the cervix has risen higher into the vagina, making it harder to locate. Following ovulation the cervix returns to its former state, positioned lower, and feels firmer with the os closed. Checking the position and consistency of the cervix, along with the cervical mucus method, can easily be performed by either partner. Women are encouraged to observe and record mood changes and breast tenderness which usually occur in the latter part of the cycle. She may be aware of ovulation pain (known as **mittelschmerz**) and/or mid cycle bleeding. All these indicators help to confirm changes in the cycle.

2: Natural family planning methods: fertility awareness

Disadvantages

❖ Requires motivation
❖ Needs to be taught by a specialist in natural family planning
❖ Requires daily commitment.

Advantages

❖ Detects beginning and end of fertile phase
❖ Can be used to promote pregnancy
❖ Higher contraceptive efficacy than any other single natural family planning method.

SELF ASSESSMENT QUESTIONS

Answers and discussion at the end of the chapter.

1. What sort of problems with the natural family planning method do you think your client may encounter?
2. How would you help your clients solve these problems?
3. For whom do you think this method might be unsuitable and why?

THE PERSONAL CONTRACEPTIVE SYSTEM

Persona is the first personal contraceptive system, under the control of the woman, which identifies when a woman is fertile. With careful and consistent use Persona is between 93 and 97% effective in preventing pregnancy; the efficacy stated is the result of ongoing prospective research which commenced in 1995 (Fig. 2.4).

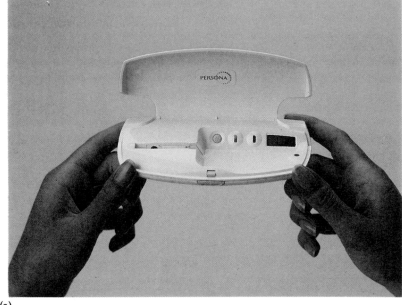

(a)

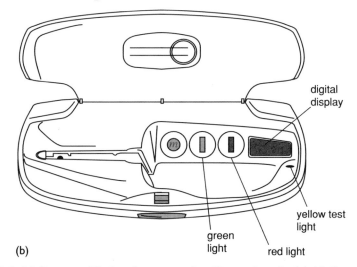

(b)

Fig. 2.4 (a) Persona (b) showing operation (Reproduced with kind permission of Unipath Ltd.)

Persona monitors (through a database) luteinizing hormone and oestrone-3-glucuronide (a metabolite of oestradiol). By testing her urine through urinary test sticks, information is given to her database which is interpreted telling her whether she is fertile or not. Persona tells a woman when the fertile period commences and ends through a system of lights: a green light indicates she is safe to have sexual intercourse; a red light indicates she should abstain or use a barrier method of contraception (this is usually 6–10 days each cycle). A yellow light indicates that she should perform a urine test to give the database more information. A urine test should be performed on an early morning urine sample and then inserted into the machine. Usually this needs to be performed eight days a month, but in the first month it will need to be done 16 days of the month to provide the database with information about a woman.

Persona can be bought over the counter at a cost of £49.95 for the starter pack and a further £9.95 each month for test sticks. A care line has been instituted by Unipath for women with fully trained staff on Persona so that advice may be given on any problems she has with this method. The telephone line is open 7am–6pm weekdays and 9am–12 midday at weekends.

Disadvantages

❖ Expensive

❖ Can only be used by women whose menstrual cycle falls within the range of 23–35 days

❖ Does not protect against sexually transmitted diseases or **human immuno-deficiency virus** (HIV).

Advantages

❖ No systemic effects

❖ Under the control of the woman

❖ Can be used to plan pregnancy

❖ Easily reversed.

Absolute contraindications

❖ Not suitable for women whose menstrual cycle does not fall in the range of 23–35 days

❖ Not suitable for women breast feeding

❖ Not suitable for women using hormone treatments

❖ Unsuitable for women with kidney or liver disease

❖ Unsuitable for women with menopausal symptoms

❖ Unsuitable for women with polycystic ovarian syndrome.

THE FERTILITY AWARENESS KIT

The fertility awareness kit is designed to teach the sympto-thermal method. It contains a video, a digital thermometer and a book of charts. This kit is available from the Family Planning Association by mail order for £19.99.

THE FUTURE

With the implementation of the personal contraceptive system there may in the future be further developments in natural family planning, but at present Persona is the latest advance.

Case History

A 51-year-old woman consulted having used natural family planning all her fertile life. She had used no other contraceptive method and had had three planned pregnancies. She was finding it difficult to identify when ovulation was occurring and was finding long periods of abstinence unsatisfactory.

Following discussion with the woman, she agreed that she and her partner would use condoms and she would continue with natural family planning. She decided that a diaphragm would stop her being able to use the natural family planning method as the use of a spermicide would affect the detecting of changes in the cervical mucus.

SELF ASSESSMENT QUESTIONS

Answers and discussion at the end of the chapter.

4. Which day of a woman's menstrual cycle is counted as the first day?

5. If a woman has a regular cycle of 5/35 days, when is she most likely to be fertile?

6. If a woman has a regular cycle of 3/21 days, when is she most likely to be fertile?

SEXUALITY AND ANXIETIES

Women who choose natural family planning methods as a contraceptive or as a means of becoming pregnant can find this method empowering; it gives them control of their lives and gives information about their body that is often concealed from them. As a method it gives men and women permission to investigate and touch a woman's body. Sometimes when a woman tries this method she finds that her cycle is not as regular as she first thought, leading to longer periods of abstinence than initially anticipated (Flynn, 1996). However, it may be argued that periodic abstinence can enhance a relationship, giving women and their partners time to enjoy a non-penetrative sexual relationship creating greater understanding of each other (Ryder & Campbell, 1995).

For women who choose this method it can be empowering; freedom of choice allows this. However, for some women for moral or religious reasons this is the only acceptable method; this can feel very limiting and unsatisfactory. If a woman has experienced unwanted or several pregnancies there may be anxiety about becoming pregnant again in the future, and it may be a good time to discuss this method and whether another method may be more suitable.

If either member of the couple has anxieties with this method – perhaps a partner does not want another pregnancy, or if used as a means of promoting pregnancy then a partner may feel a pressure to 'perform' – this may manifest itself with sexual dysfunction. Some male clients who feel a pressure to 'perform' may complain of loss of libido or erectile problems. Women who are anxious about becoming pregnant may complain of loss of libido and lack of sexual enjoyment. These problems may be very difficult for the client to discuss, but it is important that during the consultation you listen to the feelings in yourself that are evoked by the consultation, e.g. anger, sadness, as these will help you to try to understand how your client feels about the situation and whether they may wish to be referred for psychosexual counselling.

2: Natural family planning methods: fertility awareness

ANSWERS TO SELF ASSESSMENT QUESTIONS

1. **What sort of problems with the natural family planning method do you think your client may encounter?**

   Your client may encounter problems locating her cervix or may find it difficult to distinguish between the changes in the cervical mucus. She may find it difficult to remember to take her temperature every day at the same time, especially if she has young children or works shifts.

   If she is unwell or has had a disturbed sleep pattern then this will affect her basal body temperature. Events like late night parties, children waking in the night and alcohol consumption will all affect the BBT. If your client's cycle has been affected by a change in hormone levels and she has secondary amenorrhoea, for example following pregnancy or at the menopause, she may find it difficult to interpret her fertile phase, and another method may be more appropriate.

2. **How would you solve these problems?**

   If your client has difficulty locating her cervix then she will need to be taught. She may find it easier to feel her cervix if she uses a squatting position or in a standing position with one foot on a chair, and if she tries feeling in her infertile phase when the cervix is lower and easier to feel.

   If there are problems distinguishing between the changes in the cervical mucus then it is important to eliminate vaginal infection which would camouflage normal discharge. Your client may lack confidence and knowledge in her mucus changes, it may be a good idea to book more frequent consultations so that you can check the cervical mucus together throughout her cycle.

Difficulty remembering temperature taking may be solved with an alarm. A digital thermometer may be useful as it only takes 45 seconds to record the temperature, and if a mother is rushing out of bed for a crying child this may be a suitable compromise. The problem may signify the woman's dissatisfaction with the method, and another method may be more suitable.

3. **For whom do you think this method might be unsuitable and why?**

   Women who have a delay in ovulation caused by secondary amenorrhoea following childbirth or the menopause would need to have long periods of abstinence, which makes this method unsuitable for these women.

   Other women who would be considered unsuitable for this method are women who do not want to get pregnant and require a contraceptive with a high efficacy. The method would be unsuitable for women where pregnancy would be detrimental to her health or that of the foetus, e.g. following administration of a live vaccine when teratogenesis is a risk.

4. **Which day of a woman's menstrual cycle is counted as the first day?**

   The first day of a woman's menstrual cycle is counted as the first day of her period. Many women think that the first day of their cycle is at the end of their period.

5. **If a woman has a regular menstrual cycle of 5/35 days, when is she most likely to be fertile?**

   A woman ovulates between 12 and 16 days before her next period, therefore a woman with a regular 35-day cycle would be fertile between days 19 and 23 of her cycle.

6. **If a woman has a regular menstrual cycle of 3/21 days, when is she most likely to be fertile?**

   A woman with a regular 21-day cycle would be fertile between days 5 and 8 of her cycle.

MALE METHODS

- ❖ **Introduction**
- ❖ **Coitus interruptus**
- ❖ **Condoms**
- ❖ **Male sterilization**
- ❖ **Future male contraception**

3

INTRODUCTION

The choice of contraception available to a man is limited compared with that available to a woman. Most research has been aimed at female clients because it is the woman who will become pregnant and because it is easier to stop a monthly ovulation rather than a continuous sperm process. However with increasing education and sexual openness more men are taking a keen interest in this area, as shown by the number of men opting for sterilization. Health education councils and the media have tried to promote the use of the male condom in the prevention against sexually transmitted diseases and HIV with limited effect; there is still the belief that 'it won't happen to me', and as long as this exists the widespread use of condoms is impeded.

COITUS INTERRUPTUS

History and introduction

Coitus interruptus is where a man withdraws his penis from the vagina before ejaculating during sexual intercourse. It is the oldest method of contraception being referred to in the Bible (Genesis 38: verse 9) and the Koran. Coitus interruptus is widely accepted and used in Muslim and Christian communities as a method of contraception. The name coitus interruptus is rarely used by men and women – instead it is usually referred to as withdrawal, although there are many other euphemisms such as 'being careful' or 'he looks after things'. This can lead to misunderstanding during consultations if you are unaware of the euphemisms used for coitus interruptus as these can vary in different areas. You may have to clarify with the client what they are practising as a method of contraception to enable you to help them during the consultation.

Explanation of the method

This is where the man withdraws his penis before ejaculating from the woman's vagina.

Efficacy

The efficacy of coitus interruptus is variable but it can with careful and consistent use be as high as 96% effective in preventing pregnancy. However, the figure may be as low as 81% with less careful and committed use (Clubb & Knight, 1996). Another reason why this method may fail is the presence of sperm in pre-ejaculate.

Advantages

❖ Easily available
❖ Requires no clinic appointment
❖ Acceptable to certain religions
❖ No financial cost
❖ Under the control of the couple.

Disadvantages

❖ Low efficacy
❖ No protection against HIV and other sexually transmitted diseases.
❖ May inhibit enjoyment during sexual intercourse.

Absolute contraindication

❖ Men with erectile problems such as premature ejaculation.

Decision of choice

Many couples choose to use this method because of its accessibility. This may be because they have no other contraception available at the time of intercourse or because they feel that other choices are unsuitable. Coitus interruptus is often chosen as a method by couples for its religious acceptability. It may also be used initially in a new sexual relationship or where other methods seem unacceptable to the couple.

Problems encountered

❖ Pregnancy
❖ Sexual frustration
❖ Anxiety over method.

Sexuality and anxieties

You may encounter anxiety by either partner. The man may feel anxious over the responsibility placed upon him to successfully withdraw his penis before ejaculation. This may reduce his enjoyment during sexual intercourse and may lead to erectile problems. The woman may experience anxiety over her partner's ability to use withdrawal and the risk of pregnancy; as a result she may complain of loss of satisfaction during intercourse.

For many couples this may be a highly acceptable form of contraception which is under their influence and easily reversible. They have the power to revoke their decision and have 'unprotected' sexual intercourse if they wish to conceive at any time.

CONDOMS

History and introduction

Condoms were one of the first forms of contraception invented. They were made of many unusual materials and initially were seen as a protection against sexually transmitted diseases rather than pregnancy. Egyptian men were first reported to use condoms to protect themselves against infection back in 1350–1220 BC. Later in AD 1564 an Italian anatomist called Gabrielle Fallopius proclaimed to have invented a condom made of linen in an effort to protect against syphilis. During Casanova's era in the 1700s condoms were being used not only to protect against infection but also pregnancy. In the past condoms have been made of animal's bladders, oiled silk, paper and leather (Durex 1993).

With the discovery of the **acquired immune deficiency syndrome** (AIDS) in 1981 (Conor & Kingman, 1988) condoms have been widely advertised and promoted. They can be bought in supermarkets, petrol stations and vending machines and are available in public male and female toilets.

Condoms are a highly effective method and one of the few contraceptives available to a man. They are often referred to under a variety of names such as sheath, johnny, rubber and french letter.

In 1996 a new condom (Stuttaford, 1996) was released onto the market. Marketed under the name Topaz, it was invented by an engineer called Keith Jones. The Topaz aims to solve problems which men experience with the application of condom and breakages.

Explanation of method

A condom is made from a latex sheath which is applied and covers the length of an erect penis. It is disposable and should only be used once, and comes in a variety of colours and features. A condom acts as a barrier preventing sperm and ovum from meeting and pregnancy occurring.

Efficacy

The efficacy of the condom is variable – with careful and consistent use it can be as high as 98% or as low as 85%. The lower efficacy is more likely to occur in men and women who are younger and more fertile with less experience using this method (Trussell *et al.*, 1994).

3: Male methods

Disadvantages

- ❖ Perceived as messy
- ❖ Perceived as interrupting sexual intercourse
- ❖ Requires forward planning
- ❖ Loss of sensitivity
- ❖ Cannot be used in conjunction with oil-based lubricants.

Advantages

- ❖ Under the control of the couple
- ❖ No systemic effects
- ❖ Easily available
- ❖ Protection against sexually transmitted diseases and HIV
- ❖ May protect against cervical neoplasia.

Contraindications

- ❖ Allergy to latex or spermicide
- ❖ Erectile problems such as failure to maintain an erection.

Range of condoms

Condoms now come in a variety of colours, flavours and shapes. Condoms have to conform to the British Standards Institution specification (BS 3704 1989) and by June 1998 condoms sold in the European community must conform to the new single European condom standard and will have the European CE mark. Condoms will carry the BSI kitemark and the European Standard logo to ensure they have met these requirements. The use of the BSI kitemark shows that a condom complies with a recognized standard of quality and reliability. Table 3.1 lists the main varieties of kitemarked condoms available in the UK. Colours available include: gold, transparent, black, red, blue, coral, yellow, orange and green. Flavours include: mint flavoured, strawberry, banana and tangerine. Shapes include: contoured, flared, plain ended, straight and ribbed.

Decision of choice

For many men and women condoms are a convenient and easily accessible form of contraception. They allow men to share and take the responsibility for preventing pregnancy. Condoms can increase enjoyment by giving permission to men and women to touch and explore the penis. The application of a condom can be shared by either partner, creating equality in the relationship.

For many clients choosing this method may be sudden spur of the moment decision. It is often used initially in a sexual relationship, and these clients are usually younger. Many men and women prefer to use condoms to protect themselves against HIV; however there is still the belief that 'it won't happen to me'.

Table 3.1 Main varieties of kitemarked condoms available in the UK. Reproduced with kind permission of the Family Planning Association

Manufacturer & product	Presentation
LRC Products (Durex)	
All produced from hypoallergenic latex	
Spermicidally lubricated	
Elite	transparent, straight-sided, teat end, lightweight
Featherlite	transparent, straight-sided, teat end, ultra-thin
Extra Safe	coral, anatomically-shaped, teat end
Safe Play	transparent, straight-sided, teat end
Non-spermicidally lubricated	
Select	selection of coloured, ribbed and flavoured, straight-sided, teat end
Ultra Strong	transparent, straight-sided, plain end, stronger/thicker
Gossamer	transparent, straight-sided, teat end
Mates Healthcare (Mates)	
Spermicidally lubricated	
Natural	transparent, anatomically-shaped, teat end
Variety	selection of coloured, ribbed and natural; ribbed and coloured, straight-sided, natural anatomically-shaped, all teat end
Ultrasafe	transparent, anatomically-shaped, teat end
Ribbed	transparent, straight-sided, teat end, ribbed surface
Non-spermicidally lubricated	
Conform	transparent, anatomically-shaped, tighter fit, teat end
Superstrong	transparent, straight-sided, teat end, stronger/thicker
Sime Health (Jiffi)	
All produced from hypoallergenic latex	
Spermicidally lubricated	
Gold	transparent, straight-sided, teat end
Silhouette	transparent, straight-sided, teat end
Non-spermicidally lubricated	
Classic	transparent, straight-sided, teat end
Rainbow	coloured, straight-sided, teat end
Cocktail	transparent, flavoured, straight-sided, teat end
Flavours	coloured, transparent, straight-sided, teat end
Forget Me Not (produced for FP Sales Ltd)	transparent, straight-sided, teat end

3: Male methods

Table 3.1 (continued)	
Manufacturer & product	**Presentation**
Safex Supplies (Safex)	
Spermicidally lubricated	
Natural	transparent, straight-sided, teat end
Sensitive	transparent, straight-sided, teat end
Fantasy Ribbed	transparent, ribbed, anatomically-shaped, teat end
Non-spermicidally lubricated	
Natural Non-Spermicidal	transparent, straight-sided, teat end
Safe Guard Forte	transparent, straight-sided, teat end
Mr Condom (Mr Condom)	
Spermicidally lubricated	
Ribbed	transparent, straight-sided, teat end, ribbed surface
Dotted	transparent, straight-sided, teat end, dotted surface
Strong	transparent, straight-sided, teat end
Extra Fine	transparent, straight-sided, teat end, lightweight
Non-spermicidally lubricated	
Flavours	transparent, straight-sided, teat end, flavoured
Boots the Chemist (Boots)	
Spermicidally lubricated	
Extra	transparent, anatomically-shaped, teat end
Ultra Fine	transparent, straight-sided, teat end, lightweight
Motech SAM	
Spermicidally lubricated	
Topaz	transparent, straight-sided, teat end, lightweight includes soft plastic applicator ring

In The Durex Report 1994 46% of people questioned did not believe that they would contract HIV and 43% of men and women between the ages of 18 and 24 had had unprotected sexual intercourse in the last year (Durex, 1994). Research confirms (de Vincenzi, 1994) (Saracco *et al.*, 1993) that condoms used in heterosexual relationships are highly effective in preventing the transmission of HIV. Many women are now using a condom for practising safer sex and another method of contraception for the prevention of pregnancy, a practice known as the 'double Dutch'. However this is still an area that requires increased awareness and promotion.

Choosing a condom these days may be fraught with indecision for clients. How do they know which one to try? What's the difference? You are in a prime position to advise about how to use condoms, and how to help your clients choose the condom most suitable for them.

There is no legal age limit requirement which restricts the sale of condoms,

3: Male methods

which gives condoms both a wide and young user age range. Many men and women stop using condoms because of complaints of loss of sensitivity. Often change to another method is exacerbated by a user failure such as burst condom or condom coming off during sexual intercourse.

It is believed that one reason why men complain of loss of sensitivity with condoms is because they are too tight. Flared and contoured condoms are designed to give more space to the head of the penis, thus alleviating this problem. Contoured condoms are anatomically shaped to hug the glans, so that they are less likely to slip off whilst still increasing sensitivity. Ribbed condoms are straight condoms with extra bands of latex which are designed to heighten sensitivity for a woman. Straight condoms come in designs with or without a teat (the teat is to retain ejaculate). Condoms with teats such as straight, flared or contoured should be used for internal lubrication. Internal lubrication, or 'gel charging', involves putting water-soluble lubricant into the teat of the condom. As the gel liquefies around the glans, sensitivity increases.

The Topaz condom (Fig. 3.1) has been designed with an applicator, so that it unrolls the right way onto the penis, avoiding condom breakages. Topaz's applicator ensures that there is less contact with the condom, which reduces the risk of tearing the condom with fingernails and jewellery. It is sold in packs of two in discreetly designed cases and refills of six condoms are available. Each Topaz sits in its own tray and has a foil lid which should be peeled off for use. The condom should be held between the thumb and the forefinger to expel any air and placed on an erect penis with one hand. With the other hand the applicator of the Topaz condom should be held, and the condom and applicator should be eased over the penis. The purity seal of the applicator will break, allowing the applicator to pass over the penis. The condom and the applicator should be applied to the base of the penis. The applicator should be removed sideways once the condom has been fully unrolled. After the man has ejaculated, and withdrawn his penis from the vagina, the Topaz should be removed and placed in its tray. The white and green trays can be clipped together to provide a closed unit. The Topaz and its case should then be disposed of carefully. As this unit cannot be flushed down a toilet it will be applauded by environmentalists. Topaz is the only condom to incorporate details about emergency contraception in its instruction leaflet.

Condoms vary in strength. The strongest are condoms like Mates superstrong and Durex Ultrastrong, which are thicker. They are suitable for men who experience premature ejaculation or wish for other reasons to delay ejaculation. Thicker condoms are more suitable for anal intercourse, which requires the use of extra water-based lubricants. Other stronger condoms suitable for anal intercourse which are imported are HT special, Gay Safe and Hot Rubber. These should also carry the CE marking. The female condom may be used for anal intercourse if the inner ring is removed. Although male and female condoms make anal intercourse safer against sexually transmitted diseases (STDs) and HIV they are not manufactured for this use. Condoms which are thinner are designed to increase sensitivity but clients need to be aware of the need to apply these carefully: examples of these are Durex Elite or Featherlite.

Many condoms contain the spermicide Nonoxynol 9 which may give increased local irritation. There is concern over reports of local trauma caused by

3: Male methods

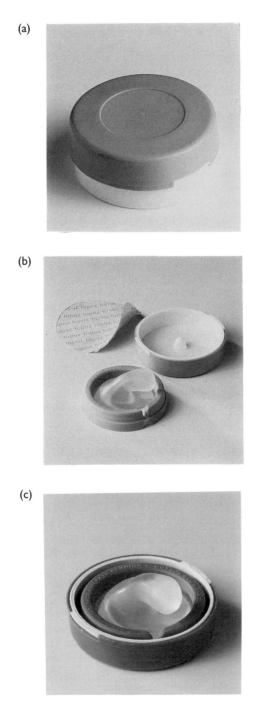

Fig. 3.1 Topaz condom (a) with applicator (b) in tray prior to use (c) in case. (Reproduced with kind permission of Motech Sam.)

Nonoxynol 9 and whether this causes vulnerability to HIV transmission (Bird, 1991) (see section on spermicides, p. 83). If a partner complains of local irritation to a condom then a condom using a non-spermicidal lubricant should be used, once genitourinary infections have been excluded.

Flavoured condoms are suitable for oral intercourse and come in a variety of flavours and colours, as already described. Condoms are available in discrete packaging aimed at different age groups.

Loss of efficacy of the condom

Various preparations affect the efficacy of the condom. These include all oil-based products including:

arachis oil enemas	fungilin	nystan cream
baby oil	gyno-daktarin	nystavescent
bath oil	gyno-pevaryl	orthodienoestrol
body oil	hair conditioner	orthogynest
butter	ice cream	pimafucin cream
cold cream	lipstick	premarin
cooking oil	low-fat spreads	skin softener
cream	massage oil	sultrin
cyclogest	monistat	vaseline
ecostatin	nizoral	witepsol-based suppositories

Teaching how to use a condom

Teaching clients how to use and apply a condom requires little time, yet may prevent user failure. Research indicates that condom breakages are more common in young and inexperienced clients (Sparrow & Lavill, 1994). Other condom failures were where the condom slipped off inside the vagina following loss of erection after sexual intercourse. Condom mishaps are most likely to occur at the beginning of a relationship (UK Family Planning Research Network, 1993) and decrease as the relationship continues. This means that new and transient relationships are most at risk of unprotected sexual intercourse.

All this information shows how important it is to teach clients how to use condoms. When teaching your clients it is helpful to show how to apply a condom using a condom demonstrator. Encourage your client to check that the condom packet has not expired and has the BSI kitemark and CE logo. When opening the condom packet clients should push the condom out of the way to avoid tearing; the condom packet should then be squeezed helping the condom to slip out. A condom should be applied before the penis comes into contact with the vulva. The condom should be placed on the erect penis and unrolled carefully along the whole length of it. Using their other hand the client should squeeze the condom at the head of the penis to expel any air. Once ejaculation has taken place the penis should be withdrawn holding the condom onto the base of the penis to ensure that it is not left in the vagina. Condoms should only be used once (Fig. 3.2) and disposed of carefully.

You should discuss with your client the loss of efficacy caused by oil-based lubricants, and given up-to-date information on condoms. As all methods of

3: Male methods

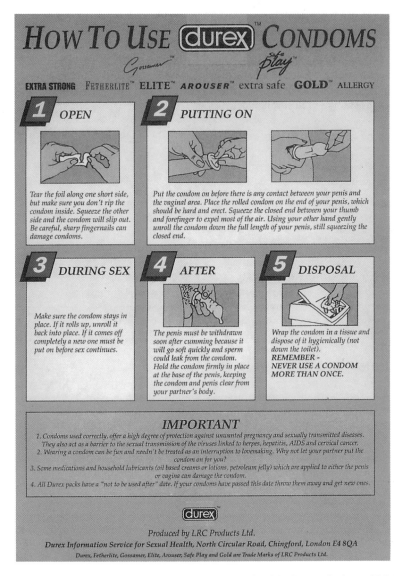

Fig. 3.2 How to use a condom. (Reproduced with kind permission of LRC Products Ltd, London.)

contraception have a failure rate it is important to discuss emergency contraception. Younger women have been found to be more likely to seek emergency contraception than older women following a condom failure (UK Family Planning Research Network, 1993); this may be for a number of reasons. However there are still large gaps in men's and women's knowledge of post-coital contraception, so this is a good time to correct misconceptions.

ACTIVITY
Practise applying condoms with either a condom demonstrator or your fingers. Do you know what condoms are available where you work?

Problems encountered

There are a number of accidents that can be encountered whilst using condoms.

❖ *THE CONDOM BURST OR SPLIT DURING SEXUAL INTERCOURSE:*
This is usually because the client has either put the condom on inside out, or not released any air or because the condom has come into contact with a fat-soluble product, e.g. baby oil (Table 3.1) which caused the condom to break. The Topaz condom has been manufactured with a device to aid correct application of the condom hopefully stopping a condom being applied inside out.

❖ *THE CONDOM SLIPPED OFF DURING INTERCOURSE OR REMAINED INSIDE THE VAGINA WHEN THE PENIS WAS REMOVED FOLLOWING INTERCOURSE:*
This usually happens when a man loses his erection and fails to hold onto the condom when he removes his penis from the vagina leaving the condom inside the vagina. The condom can also slip off when applied inside out.

❖ *THE CONDOM WAS RIPPED WHILST IT WAS APPLIED:*
This can be due to ragged nails or rings, and a new condom should be applied if this happens.

❖ *DIFFICULTIES APPLYING THE CONDOM – 'IT'S TOO SMALL OR TOO BIG':*
Condoms can now be bought to accommodate different sizes of penis. All condoms are able to expand so should not be too small. However Mates now make condoms in contoured and flared shapes; flared are suitable for men who complain that the condom is too small and contoured for men who find condoms too big. Durex also make a condom called 'Surefit' for men who want smaller sized condoms.

❖ *ALLERGY TO THE CONDOM:*
Men who complain of allergy to condoms are usually allergic to the spermicide and should try a condom which does not contain a spermicide; all condoms are hypoallergenic.

❖ *LOSS OF SENSITIVITY:*
Condoms which are plain ended and thin will help increase sensitivity. Couples can also try 'gel charging' which involves putting a small amount of

water-soluble lubricant into the condom with a teat before application; this can also increase sensitivity. Many men complain of loss of sensitivity because the condom is too tight; flared condoms may help alleviate this problem.

Case History

A 33-year-old married woman consulted concerned that she had a condom left inside her vagina. The condom was found and removed from the vagina. During the session the nurse asked whether emergency contraception was wanted, and whether the woman was happy with her method of contraception.

The woman was trying to conceive, but explained that the condom was from another partner and she would therefore want emergency contraception. As she had already had unprotected sexual intercourse with her regular partner with whom she was trying to conceive throughout her cycle, and was now beyond the limits for emergency contraception, this was contraindicated. The risks of this episode of unprotected sexual intercourse were discussed in relation to pregnancy and genitourinary infection. A pregnancy test was performed which was negative and a further test was arranged for a week's time when the client's next period was due.

SELF ASSESSMENT QUESTIONS

Answers and discussion at the end of the chapter.

1. What sort of condom would you recommend for anal intercourse?
2. What is gel charging?
3. Name ten products which will cause condoms to burst.

The future

In the future any condom that reduces condom breakages or has a higher efficacy is likely to receive a warm welcome. A new polyurethane condom will be available which is less likely to be affected by fat-soluble products, and has the advantages of being stronger and more durable.

Sexuality and anxieties

There are many different perceptions regarding the use of condoms. Studies in the USA have shown (Grady *et al.*, 1993) that many men believe that using a condom 'shows you care', however at the same time it may give other messages, e.g. 'that you have AIDS' or 'that you think that your partner has AIDS'. These anxieties cause a dilemma for men and women, and illustrate how difficult it is to talk to a new partner about sexual intercourse and safer sex. The embarrassment this causes may be the reason why so many couples have unprotected sexual intercourse. Men and women often consult following accidents with condoms for emergency contraception. New relationships appear to be the riskiest time for condom breakages (UK Family Planning Research Network, 1993). However research with commercial sex workers in the USA (Albert *et al.*, 1995) suggests that regular condom use leads to the development of techniques which reduce breakage and slippage of condoms. When clients consult for emergency contraception following a condom breakage this is a prime opportunity to discuss condom technique and alleviate any future problems. Many men and women use a condom breakage as their reason for requiring emergency contraception when in fact they have had unprotected sexual intercourse which they feel will be disapproved of by professionals. This makes it difficult to obtain accurate statistics for condom use and breakage.

Condoms give a man the opportunity to take part in contraception, they are often used at some point in a relationship, and have the advantage of taking care of the 'mess'. However for some women this may be the very reason why they dislike condoms; the 'mess' or ejaculate may be warm and exciting.

Condoms can give a woman permission to touch her partner's penis; she can use a condom as part of a safe form of foreplay by applying it herself or together with her partner. This can give couples the opportunity to talk about their sexual needs and desires.

MALE STERILIZATION

History and introduction

Male sterilization has become a popular choice of permanent contraception for many couples; the surgical procedure is known as a vasectomy. The first experiments into occlusion of the vas deferens were conducted as early as 1830 by Sir Astley Cooper, and later in the twentieth century with advancement of surgery and anaesthesia, vasectomies became available to men. This resulted in the Family Planning Association opening its first vasectomy clinic in October 1968.

Explanation of the method

A vasectomy involves cutting the vas deferens, which is the tube that transports sperm from the epididymis in the testes to the seminal vesicles. By cutting the vas deferens sperm is unable to be ejaculated and a man will become infertile once the vas deferens is clear of sperm, which takes about 3 months.

Efficacy

A vasectomy is a highly effective form of contraception. Its immediate failure rate is 1 in 1000; the late failure rate is between 1 in 3000 and 1 in 7000 (Belfield, 1997).

Disadvantages

❖ Alternative contraception is required until two consecutive clear sperm counts are obtained
❖ Surgical procedure required
❖ Local or general anaesthesia required
❖ Not easily reversible.

Advantages

❖ Permanent method
❖ High efficacy
❖ Removal of anxiety of unplanned pregnancy
❖ Safe and simple procedure.

Absolute contraindications

❖ Serious physical disability
❖ Urological problems
❖ Relationship problems
❖ Indecision by either partner.

Range of method

During a vasectomy the vas deferens will be cut and either cautery or a ligature will be applied. Part of the incised vas deferens may be sent to pathology to confirm that the correct tube has been cut. Each end of the vas deferens will be buried in separate tissue layers to prevent them rejoining (see Fig 3.3).

Side effects

❖ Infection
❖ Haematoma
❖ Sperm granuloma.

Counselling a couple for a vasectomy

Vasectomy counselling is preferably performed with both partners, as this is a decision which will permanently affect both parties. As this is a permanent method of contraception the couple should be sure of their decision, and aware that this is very difficult to reverse. Couples during counselling are often asked to consider certain scenarios, e.g. how they would feel if their partner died, would they want to have children with someone else? Or if one of their children died, would they want to have more? If they have not had children is there a likelihood

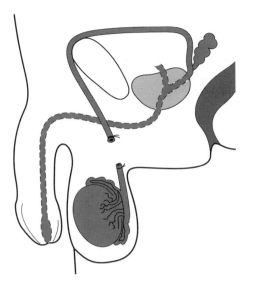

Fig. 3.3 Male sterilization. (Reproduced from Women's Sexual Health, G. Andrews (ed.), 1996, Baillière Tindall.)

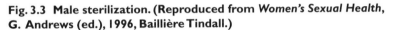

they will change their mind? Sometimes clients have not considered major life events and their effects, and during counselling decide to delay such a permanent decision.

Men are often concerned about their ability to maintain erections and have sexual intercourse following a vasectomy. You can advise your clients that a vasectomy does not affect libido or erections and their ejaculate will look the same except it will no longer contain sperm, which is not detectable to the human eye.

It is important that your client continues to use an effective form of contraception, as it may cause considerable distress if a client has a vasectomy and then finds his partner is pregnant. Contraception will be required for about 3 months following a vasectomy. Once two consecutive negative sperm counts have been obtained then the use of another form of contraception may be ceased.

There has been concern over an increased incidence of testicular (West, 1992) and prostrate cancer (Giovannucci et al., 1993a,b) in men who have had a vasectomy. At the moment there is no definite proof of a link between cancer of the prostrate or testes and vasectomies (FPA, 1993; National Institutes of Health, 1993); if there is it is very small. It may be that men who have had a vasectomy are more aware and consult earlier if they notice a problem (Howards & Peterson, 1993). Smoking increases the risk of all cancers, including testicular and prostrate cancer. Cancer of the prostrate is a disease found in older men; 90% of all deaths from cancer of the prostrate occur after the age of 65.

Vasectomies can fail even after negative sperm counts and it is important to discuss this with your client beforehand (Brahams, 1995). This is thought to be due to re-canalization of the vas deferens.

Procedure

A vasectomy may be performed under local or general anaesthetic. One or two incisions are performed on each scrotum so that the vas deferens may be located, excised and ligated.

Post vasectomy

Men should be encouraged to take things gently as this will reduce the risk of bruising. They should wear a scrotal support and avoid heavy lifting, strenuous exercise and sexual intercourse for a week post operatively. Pain may be eased by the use of ice packs and analgesia; frozen peas are suitable for this purpose as they mould around the area well, reducing swelling and pain. A follow-up study of men who had had a vasectomy (Canter & Goldthorpe, 1995) found that the median time to full recovery after the operation was 7 days. Many clients do not allow enough time for full recovery, which increases their chances of getting post-operative complications.

Once a man has had two consecutive sperm tests which are clear of sperm then he can stop using another form of contraception. It takes about 3 months for a man's ejaculate to clear of sperm.

Following a vasectomy a man should watch for any signs of infection, haematoma and sperm granuloma. Any signs of rising temperature and/or pain or swelling around the testes may indicate infection, which will need to be treated with antibiotics. A haematoma is likely to happen if a client has not given himself enough time to recuperate; it should be treated with ice packs, analgesia and rest. A sperm granuloma can cause pain and localized swelling but can also be asymptomatic; it occurs when sperm leaks into the surrounding tissue where the vas deferens was excised and may need further excision.

Reversal of a vasectomy

Reversal is often requested when a man has commenced a new relationship and wishes to have children. Reversal of a vasectomy is easier to perform than reversal of a female sterilization. However it may only be 50% successful in achieving a pregnancy (this may be higher in skilled hands), and may be lower if the

3: Male methods

SELF ASSESSMENT QUESTIONS

Answers and discussion at the end of the chapter.
4. Roughly how long does it take for a man to achieve a negative sperm count following a vasectomy?
5. What advantages do you think a vasectomy has over female sterilization?
6. What anxieties may a man have over a vasectomy?

Do you know what facilities are available locally for men requesting a vasectomy? Is there a waiting list? What are your clients told about after care, are you giving the same information?

operation was performed more than 10 years ago. When reversing a vasectomy the vas deferens is re-anastomosed, which may be successful, but there is a risk that anti-sperm antibodies will develop and cause the sperm count to be low, making pregnancy difficult to achieve.

Sexuality and anxieties

Vasectomies have become more fashionable in recent times, which coincides with the 'sharing caring image' of 'new men'. However sometimes it can be used as an emotional weapon – women may say 'it's his turn to do something now', which may cause conflict in the future in their relationship. There can be an element of self-sacrifice and martyrdom about the decision, which is why meeting both parties at the counselling session may help to bring this into the open for discussion.

A vasectomy may be chosen following completion of a family but also may be the result of an unplanned pregnancy, which may scare a couple into making a decision.

After a vasectomy some men may experience signs of grief over their loss of fertility and sexuality. This will depend on how the man feels about his decision; if he feels forced or coerced into the decision then he may feel anger and sadness over his loss. Some men see a vasectomy as tantamount to castration, and have anxieties that their ability to function as a man will be impaired permanently. Many men see a vasectomy as their opportunity to do something, especially after their partner has had children. This can cement their relationship and bring them closer, reducing anxiety over further pregnancy.

FUTURE MALE CONTRACEPTION

Research is currently being undertaken into male hormonal contraception containing testosterone and progestogen. Weekly injections of testosterone enanthate 200 mg has been shown to produce azoospermia in about two-thirds of men within 3 months and severe oligospermia in the remaining men (Bonn, 1996). However trials are being commenced on testosterone bucyclate which offers the advantage of longer-term contraception requiring one injection every 3–4 months.

Some women feel that men cannot be relied upon to be responsible for taking a hormonal method as they do not have to suffer the long-term effects of pregnancy. However today men are increasingly interested and prepared to accept the responsibility of sharing contraception.

3: Male methods

ANSWERS TO SELF ASSESSMENT QUESTIONS

1. **What sort of condom would you recommend for anal intercourse?**

   Although condoms are not manufactured for anal intercourse the thickest condom should be used such as Durex Ultrastrong and Mates Ultra safe. A water-based lubricant should be used in conjunction with a condom with anal intercourse.

2. **What is gel charging?**

   Gel charging is also known as internal lubrication; it increases sensitivity for a man when using condoms. A small amount of water-soluble lubricant is inserted into a condom with a teat. During sexual intercourse this liquefies, increasing sensation.

3. **Name ten products which will cause condoms to burst.**

   The following products cause condoms to burst: arachis oil enemas, baby oil, bath oil, body oil, butter, cold cream, cream, cooking oil, cyclogest, ecostatin, fungilin, gynodaktarin, gyno-pevaryl, hair conditioner, ice cream, lipstick, low-fat spreads, massage oil, monistat, nizoral, nystan cream, nystavescent, orthodienoestrol, orthogynest, pimafucin cream, premarin, skin softener, sultrin, vaseline and witepsol-based suppositories.

4. **Roughly how long does it take for a man to achieve a negative sperm count following a vasectomy?**

   It takes roughly 3 months for a man to achieve a negative sperm count, and he can consider it safe to have sexual intercourse when he has had two consecutive negative sperm counts.

5. **What advantages do you think a vasectomy has over female sterilization?**

   A vasectomy can easily be performed under local anaesthetic, whilst the majority of female sterilizations are performed under general anaesthetic. Anatomically the scrotum and vas deferens are easy to locate, whilst with a woman locating the fallopian tubes is harder as they are under muscle and fat layers. This is why women may be in hospital for longer whilst a man may go home following the procedure.

6. **What anxieties may a man have over a vasectomy?**

   Men have anxieties over their ability to achieve an orgasm, maintain an erection and changes in their ejaculate. Most of their anxieties surround myths about vasectomy which include impotence and sexual dysfunction. They may also have anxieties over prostate and testicular cancer. Some men may have anxieties about the procedure and fears about what may happen.

3: Male methods

FEMALE BARRIER METHODS

4

INTRODUCTION

Contraception not only gives women protection against pregnancy, but also gives women power over their bodies. It gives women the opportunity to choose when to conceive or not, allowing them the chance to develop their lives through education and careers. However this also creates dilemmas: by having highly effective contraception women now have to decide when to conceive, and sometimes there never seems to be a right time to do this! Many women leave trying to conceive till late into their thirties, and then find they have difficulty becoming pregnant; other women have contraceptive failures which may subconsciously stem from their desire to become pregnant.

HISTORY

Contraception has changed dramatically over the last ten years with the launch of longer-term methods such as Norplant and Mirena. These methods give an excellent alternative to sterilization and offer a wider choice to all women. The female condom has given women the opportunity to practise safer sex; not only is it easily inserted but it is also available over the counter in chemists.

THE DIAPHRAGM

Introduction and history

Women have used a variety of materials as barrier methods in the past, such as oiled cloth, sponges, leaves and fruit often soaked with vinegar or lemon juice. A

German doctor named Hasse, who used the pseudonym Mesinga, is credited with the introduction of the diaphragm in 1882 which gave women greater freedom over their bodies. It was not until 1974 that all contraception was provided free of charge to men and women. Earlier, women had to give proof of marriage as contraception was not available to non-married women until the late 1960s.

Explanation of method

The diaphragm is a latex rubber dome which is inserted into the vagina (see Fig. 4.1). It covers the cervix, acting as a barrier to sperm and therefore helping to prevent pregnancy.

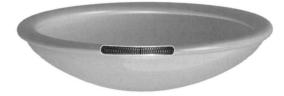

Fig. 4.1 Diaphragm. (Reproduced from _Women's Sexual Health_, G. Andrews (ed.), 1996, Baillière Tindall.)

Efficacy

With careful and consistent use the diaphragm is 92–96% effective when used with a spermicide in preventing pregnancy in the first year. With typical use where a woman does not use this method carefully the efficacy is 82–90% effective when used with a spermicide in preventing pregnancy in the first year (Bounds, 1994). Failure rates for the diaphragm depend on how effectively the woman uses it. Does she use the diaphragm for every episode of sexual intercourse? Is her cervix covered each episode? Is she using her diaphragm according to guidelines? Other factors which influence the failure rate of all methods are a woman's age and how often she is having sexual intercourse. For example if a woman is aged 40 and uses a diaphragm as a contraceptive she is less fertile than a woman aged 25 so a diaphragm is a more effective contraceptive for her.

The use of a spermicide with the diaphragm is currently recommended. The only study which compared the diaphragm with and without spermicide (Bounds _et al._, 1995) did not give significant results for the use of a diaphragm being effective if used alone. Until research proves that a diaphragm is as effective without spermicide as it is with spermicide current guidelines recommend that you teach your client to continue to use the diaphragm with a spermicide.

Disadvantages

* ❖ Requires motivation
* ❖ Needs to be used carefully and consistently for optimum efficacy

❖ Needs to be used with a spermicide which may be perceived as messy

❖ May increase the risk of cystitis and urinary tract infections

❖ No protection against HIV.

Advantages

❖ Under the control of the woman

❖ May give some protection against cervical cancer and sexually transmitted diseases

❖ No systemic side effects

❖ Provides vaginal lubrication

❖ Can be used during menstruation

❖ Gives a woman permission to touch and explore her body.

Contraindications

❖ Pregnancy

❖ Undiagnosed genital tract bleeding should be investigated and treated first

❖ Poor vaginal muscle tone or prolapse

❖ Congenital abnormality such as two cervices or septal wall defects (where the vagina is separated into two by a wall)

❖ Allergy to rubber or spermicide

❖ Present vaginal, cervical, or pelvic infection should be investigated and treated first

❖ Recurrent urinary tract infections

❖ Past history of toxic shock syndrome

❖ Women who feel unable to touch their genital area because of personal or religious reasons.

Side effects

❖ Urinary tract infection

❖ Toxic shock syndrome – associated with diaphragms being worn for more than 30 hours

❖ Vaginal irritation.

Range of method

There are three main types of diaphragm.

The flat spring diaphragm

This type of diaphragm has a flat spring in the rim of the diaphragm and is available in sizes 55–95 mm (rising in steps of 5 mm). Suitable for women with an anterior or midplane positioned cervix.

4: Female barrier methods

Coiled spring diaphragm

This type of diaphragm has a coiled spring in the rim of the diaphragm and is available in sizes 55–95 mm (rising in steps of 5 mm). This type of diaphragm is suitable for women who find a flat spring diaphragm uncomfortable either because they have strong vaginal muscles or are sensitive to vaginal pressure. It is also recommended to women with a shallow symphysis pubis.

Arcing spring diaphragm

This type of diaphragm is available in sizes 55–95 mm (rising in steps of 5 mm). This type of diaphragm is suitable for women with a posterior positioned cervix, or where a woman has difficulty feeling her cervix.

Decision of choice

The decision of the type of diaphragm you fit your client will depend on a vaginal examination. You will need to assess the vagina and cervix to exclude infection, poor muscle tone and prolapse. When examining your client to estimate the size of diaphragm required you should measure the distance from the posterior fornix (the area immediately behind the cervix) to the symphysis pubis (the bone in front of the bladder) with your fingers (Fig. 4.2). The measurement on

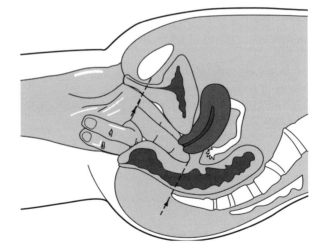

Fig. 4.2 Estimating the size of the diaphragm to be fitted. (Reproduced with kind permission from *Handbook of Family Planning*, 2nd edition, N. Loudon (ed.), 1991, Churchill Livingstone.)

your fingers corresponds to the size of diaphragm required for your client (Fig. 4.3). With practice you will find it that this is not difficult; it can be useful beforehand to measure your fingers to see where a diaphragm measures on your fingers. The diaphragm should be fitted now to check that the correct size has been

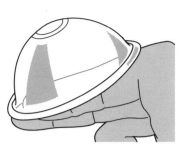

Fig. 4.3 Size of diaphragm on hand. (Reproduced with kind permission from _Handbook of Family Planning_, 2nd edition, N. Loudon (ed.), 1991, Churchill Livingstone.)

chosen (Figs 4.4 and 4.5). The diaphragm should cover the cervix and sit tucked up behind the symphysis pubis. If it protrudes into the introitus then the diaphragm is either too large (Fig. 4.6) or fitted incorrectly. If there is a gap of a finger or more then the diaphragm is too small (Fig. 4.7). Your client should be unable to feel the diaphragm _in situ_ if fitted correctly.

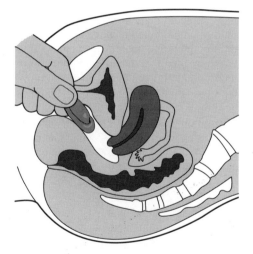

Fig. 4.4 Diaphragm being inserted. (Reproduced with kind permission from _Handbook of Family Planning_, 2nd edition, N. Loudon (ed.), 1991, Churchill Livingstone.)

How to teach a diaphragm fitting

This can feel a very threatening and embarrassing situation to your client, so it is important that your examination room is quiet, private and free from interruptions. This consultation can take some time so allow at least half an hour; you will

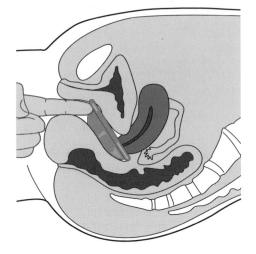

Fig. 4.5 Checking the position of the diaphragm. (Reproduced with kind permission from *Handbook of Family Planning*, 2nd edition, N. Loudon (ed.), 1991, Churchill Livingstone.)

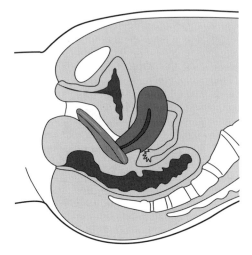

Fig. 4.6 Diaphragm too large. (Reproduced with kind permission from *Handbook of Family Planning*, 2nd edition, N. Loudon (ed.), 1991, Churchill Livingstone.)

both feel more at ease if time is not an issue. Usually a diaphragm fitting teaching session is spread over two consultations. The first visit includes initial fitting and teaching the client to locate her cervix, remove and fit the diaphragm. The second consultation includes teaching spermicidal application. Although this can be done at either visit, it is useful to have a second consultation to solve any

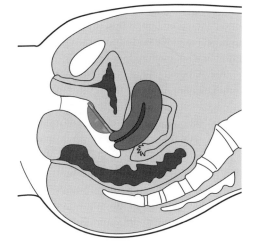

Fig. 4.7 Diaphragm too small. (Reproduced with kind permission from
Handbook of Family Planning, **2nd edition, N. Loudon (ed.), 1991, Churchill**
Livingstone.)

problems. The more comfortable your client feels the more at ease she will be in the situation and the more likely she is to succeed. Before examining your client you should show her a diaphragm and, using diagrams or a teaching model, show her how the diaphragm sits inside the vagina. Some women find this slightly difficult to understand at first, and how you approach this will vary with each client. Try and find out how much she knows and build upon this. Remember the majority of women may have never felt their cervix or have thought much about its significance. Discuss how you are going to teach your client to fit her diaphragm; this will help her feel more comfortable with the situation.

Once you have estimated the correct size of diaphragm and it is *in situ,* your client should be taught to feel inside her vagina and feel the position of the diaphragm and cervix. It is helpful if you wear a pair of gloves during this part of the consultation in case you need to help her by holding the diaphragm at some point. To teach your client she should be encouraged to wash her hands and either squat or put one foot on a chair. She should then feel inside her vagina so that she can understand how the diaphragm sits (Fig 4.8). You will now need her to feel inside her vagina. It is helpful if you give your client an idea of where her cervix is positioned, and what it feels like. The cervix has been described as a fleshy lump feeling like the end of your nose. It is important that she is able to locate her cervix, so that she is aware of it being covered by the diaphragm, to ensure efficacy.

When your client is able to locate her cervix, ask her to remove her diaphragm by putting her index finger over the anterior rim of the diaphragm and pulling downwards (Fig 4.9). The diaphragm should slip easily out. If she finds this difficult ask her to bear downwards, making removal easier. You may want to take the diaphragm and rinse it for your client so that it does not become too slippery initially for her to fit. She can insert the diaphragm by squeezing it together

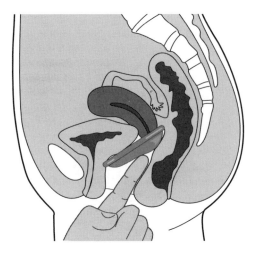

Fig. 4.8 Checking a diaphragm covering the cervix (standing position). (Reproduced with kind permission from *Handbook of Family Planning*, 2nd edition, N. Loudon (ed.), 1991, Churchill Livingstone.)

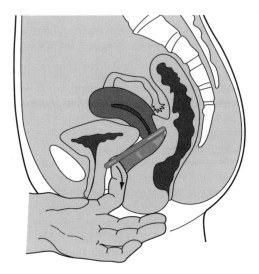

Fig. 4.9 Client removing a diaphragm (standing position). (Reproduced with kind permission from *Handbook of Family Planning*, 2nd edition, N. Loudon (ed.), 1991, Churchill Livingstone.)

firmly with one hand, or by using her thumb and second index finger to squeeze it together while her first index finger remains inside the diaphragm, giving more control over it. The diaphragm should then be inserted into the vagina as far as it will go, pushing the anterior rim of the diaphragm underneath the ledge of the symphysis pubis. Encourage your client to check that her cervix is covered, and that she feels that the diaphragm is fitted correctly. Next check by examination that your client has fitted her diaphragm correctly.

Once your client is able to locate her cervix, fit and remove her diaphragm she is able to practise using it. Usually a second consultation is made about a week later. This allows your client time to practise, whilst she uses another form of contraception to avoid pregnancy. During this time she should sleep with the diaphragm *in situ*, open her bowels, have sexual intercourse, and practise removing and fitting her diaphragm, so that if she has any problems these can be discussed and solved. Occasionally it may be necessary to combine both visits into one.

At the next visit you should advise your client to come with her diaphragm already in place. By doing this you will be able to check that she is able to fit her diaphragm correctly. This is a good time to revise care of the diaphragm, how to use spermicide and how long the diaphragm should be left *in situ*. All this information should be backed up with the appropriate leaflets, details of when your client should consult early and when a routine consultation should be carried out.

You should weigh your client at both consultations, and advise her that if her weight fluctuates by 3 kg either way she will need to have her diaphragm checked, and may require a smaller or larger diaphragm to be fitted.

The success of these consultations is very much down to the approach you give the session. If you are teaching your client to locate her cervix and she is having difficulty, if she is using a squatting position you may find that communication between you both is improved if you assume a squatting position so that you are both at the same eye level. Given time and an empathetic approach your client will gain confidence to succeed. Often clients will have problems fitting the diaphragm and locating their cervix, and may need longer at the initial consultation. Sometimes, depending on the client, you may find giving her some time by herself helpful if she feels hampered by the situation. It is important to assess each client individually; some women may require more privacy than others.

Use of the diaphragm

If your client gets into the habit of putting her diaphragm in regularly at the time she is most likely to have sexual intercourse then she is less likely to forget to put it in prior to intercourse. The diaphragm should be fitted with two 2 cm strips of spermicidal cream or gel on both sides of the diaphragm. This will give contraceptive protection for 3 hours. After 3 hours if no sexual intercourse has taken place more spermicide will need to be inserted e.g. pessary. However if sexual intercourse has taken place, and further intercourse is likely later than 3 hours after insertion, the diaphragm should be left *in situ* and additional spermicide e.g. pessary inserted into the vagina 5–10 minutes prior to intercourse to give additional cover.

The diaphragm should be left *in situ* for 6 hours after the last episode of sexual intercourse, but no longer than 24 hours to avoid the risk of toxic shock syndrome and pressure ulcers forming.

Lastly it is important to cover care of the diaphragm. It should be washed with mild soap and water and dried. Talcum powders, detergents and perfumes should be avoided as these will affect the natural flora in the vagina. The diaphragm should be bent back into shape and kept in its case following use.

The diaphragm should be kept away from direct sunlight and radiators as these may cause the diaphragm to perish. Your client should be encouraged to check her diaphragm for holes as this will reduce its effectiveness.

Preparations that reduce the efficacy of the diaphragm

The following preparations should not be used with a diaphragm as they damage the latex rubber:

arachis oil enemas	fungilin	nystan cream
baby oil	gyno-daktarin	nystavescent
bath oil	gyno-pevaryl	orthodienoestrol
body oil	hair conditioner	orthogynest
butter	ice cream	pimafucin cream
cold cream	lipstick	premarin
cooking oil	low-fat spreads	skin softener
cream	massage oil	sultrin
cyclogest	monistat	vaseline
ecostatin	nizoral	witepsol-based suppositories

Subsequent visits

You should see your client routinely every 6 months to check that the diaphragm is being fitted correctly by her and to review weight. The diaphragm should be renewed every year.

You should advise your client to return earlier if any of the following happens:

❖ Her weight varies by 3 kg

❖ Her diaphragm deteriorates, has a hole etc.

❖ The diaphragm becomes uncomfortable

❖ Pregnancy, the diaphragm should be checked following any pregnancy e.g. miscarriage, abortion, birth

❖ She has a vaginal infection. A new diaphragm should be fitted once the infection has been investigated and treated, to prevent re-infection.

SELF ASSESSMENT QUESTIONS

Answers and discussion at the end of the chapter.

1. Which preparations should not be used with a diaphragm?

2. How would you help a client who is unable to locate her cervix?

3. For which clients would an arcing diaphragm be appropriate?

Problems encountered

The following are some problems you may encounter during your consultation.

❖ *YOUR CLIENT IS UNABLE TO LOCATE HER CERVIX:*
   This can be because your client lacks confidence and needs more time. Try asking her to assume a different position, i.e. squatting or placing a foot on a chair. Sometimes you may meet a client who has regularly been using a diaphragm but has never been taught to locate her cervix.
   If your client's cervix is very posterior then it will be easier for her if you fit an arcing diaphragm. An arcing diaphragm has a spring which causes the diaphragm to fall naturally to the posterior part of the vagina

❖ *THE DIAPHRAGM DOES NOT COVER YOUR CLIENT'S CERVIX:*
   This can be because the diaphragm is too small and she needs a larger sized diaphragm or because her cervix is posterior and an arcing diaphragm is more suitable.

❖ *YOUR CLIENT FINDS HER DIAPHRAGM TOO MESSY:*
   If your client complains that the diaphragm is messy try changing her spermicide. A gel type of spermicide which is clear tends to have a more runny appearance than a cream type spermicide, or she could try foam spermicide.

❖ *YOUR CLIENT IS UNABLE TO REMOVE HER DIAPHRAGM:*
   Ask your client to bear downwards as this usually helps with removal. Remind her that the diaphragm cannot get lost. If she cannot remove it at that time then she should not panic but leave removal until she is more relaxed.

❖ *YOUR CLIENT FINDS THE DIAPHRAGM CAUSES VAGINAL IRRITATION:*
   Vaginal irritation may be due to a local sensitivity to a spermicide. Try a different spermicide. Always exclude vaginal infection by investigating first.

❖ *YOUR CLIENT COMPLAINS THAT HER PARTNER CAN FEEL THE DIAPHRAGM:*
   If your client complains that her partner can feel the diaphragm check that the diaphragm is the correct size and she is fitting it correctly. If these are not the cause of the problem and the patient's cervix is suitable then a cervical cap could be fitted.

❖ *YOUR CLIENT COMPLAINS OF RECURRENT CYSTITIS:*
   If your client complains of recurrent cystitis encourage her to empty her bladder before having sexual intercourse. Your should also check her diaphragm – it may be an incorrect size. If she has a flat spring diaphragm then changing her diaphragm to a coiled spring, which is softer, will help; or if she is suitable a cervical cap may be fitted. Research has shown that women using a diaphragm

4: Female barrier methods

were two to three times more likely to be referred with a urinary tract infection than women not using a diaphragm (Vessey, 1988), so women experiencing recurrent urine tract infections may need to review their method of contraception.

Sexuality and anxieties

A client who chooses to use a diaphragm and is successful with it can find the diaphragm gives her permission to investigate her vagina, allowing her to touch areas that may have seemed forbidden. Often women have little or no knowledge of this area of their body and have built up their own ideas about their vagina. Not only can a diaphragm act as a contraceptive, but it can educate and illuminate a hidden area.

You may find that your client complains that her diaphragm is 'messy'. This may be due to real problems with a type of spermicide but often there is an underlying problem. A client who complains that her diaphragm is messy may feel that sexual intercourse is messy. Some women have fantasies about their vagina – they feel that it is a clean, sterile area and forget that it produces its own natural discharge. They find sperm messy and as a result of these feelings there may be a problem with sexual intercourse. Given time and awareness of the feelings that the client is transferring you will find that she may talk about her anxieties. However, sometimes clients are not ready or able to look at their feelings, but may do so in the future.

Clients may panic if they are unable to remove their diaphragm. Behind this may lie the image that the diaphragm has disappeared into the midst of nowhere. Through lack of knowledge men and women can create very strong images of their bodies which can be frightening and strange.

A woman who chooses the diaphragm may do so because of its lower efficacy compared to other methods. She may have a subconscious desire to become pregnant or may actively use the method to become pregnant without letting her partner know.

THE CERVICAL CAP

Introduction and history

The cervical cap is not as widely used as the diaphragm, but in recent years it has had a renaissance. The reason why it is not as widely chosen is because it is only suitable for a certain type of cervix and because fewer family planning nurses and doctors are experienced at fitting the cervical cap and teaching clients how to use it.

Explanation of the method

There are three types of cervical cap which are made of rubber, smaller than a diaphragm, covering the cervix only and held by suction. The cervical cap helps to prevent pregnancy by acting as a barrier, stopping the sperm and ovum from meeting.

Efficacy

With careful and consistent use the cervical cap, like the diaphragm, is 92–96% effective when used with a spermicide in preventing pregnancy in the first year. With typical use where a woman does not use this method carefully the efficacy is 82–90% when used with a spermicide in preventing pregnancy in the first year (Bounds, 1994).

Disadvantages

❖ Requires motivation
❖ Needs to be used carefully and consistently for optimum efficacy
❖ Needs to be used with a spermicide which may be perceived as messy
❖ May be harder to insert and remove than a diaphragm
❖ No protection against HIV.

Advantages

❖ Under the control of the woman
❖ May give some protection against cervical cancer and sexually transmitted diseases
❖ No systemic side effects
❖ Provides vaginal lubrication
❖ Can be used during menstruation
❖ Gives a woman permission to touch and explore her body
❖ No increase in urinary symptoms and cystitis.

Contraindications

❖ Inability of the client to locate her cervix
❖ Unsuitable cervix e.g. shape, position
❖ Pregnancy
❖ Undiagnosed genital tract bleeding should be investigated first
❖ Congenital abnormality such as two cervices or septal wall defects (where the vagina is separated into two by a wall)
❖ Allergy to rubber or spermicide
❖ Present vaginal, cervical, or pelvic infection should be investigated and treated first
❖ Past history of toxic shock syndrome
❖ Women who feel unable to touch their genital area because of personal or religious reasons.

4: Female barrier methods

Range of method

There are three types of cervical cap (Fig. 4.10):

- ❖ Vault cap (Dumas cap)
- ❖ Cervical cap (Prentif cavity rim)
- ❖ Vimule cap.

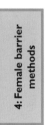

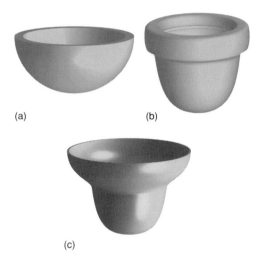

(a)   (b)

(c)

Fig. 4.10 (a) Vault cap; (b) cervical cap; (c) vimule cap. (Reproduced from
Women's Sexual Health, **G. Andrews (ed.), 1996, Baillière Tindall.)**

Decision of choice
The vault cap

The vault cap is bowl-shaped and covers the cervix by suction. It is available in
five sizes – 50 mm, 55 mm, 60 mm, 65 mm, 75 mm – labelled nos 1–5. It is suitable for women with short cervices where the rim of the vault cap will adhere to
the vault of the vagina.

The cervical cap

The cervical cap is a soft thimble-shaped cap which comes in sizes 22–31 mm rising in 3 mm steps. It is suitable for a woman with a long parallel-sided cervix; it
fits snugly over the cervix and is held there by suction. It is not suitable for
women with damaged or short cervices.

The vimule cap

The vimule is a combination of a vault and cervical cap. It is available in three
sizes – 42 mm, 48 mm and 54 mm. It has a thimble shape like the cervical cap but
has a flanged rim that, like the vault cap, adheres to the vaginal wall. The vimule
is held onto the vault of the vagina by suction.

How to teach a cap fitting

The cap is fitted in a similar way to a diaphragm. Most women who wish to use the cap have used a diaphragm previously which makes a cap fitting easier. Recently the cap has gained popularity and women often refer to it as the 'new cap'.

The cervical cap is squeezed between the thumb and two first fingers, and inserted into the vagina. Removing your thumb the cap will open and can then be guided over the cervix. Once the cap is over the cervix, check that there is no cervix outside the cap and that there is no gap around the rim of the cervix. You should be able to feel the cervix through the cap. The cervical cap is removed by inserting a finger underneath the rim of the cap. This releases the suction which holds the cap *in situ* and the cap can then be removed easily.

Once you have fitted your client with the cap, you should encourage her to feel the position of the cap and teach her to locate her cervix. It is easier for the client to fit her cap if she uses a squatting position or puts one foot on a chair. She should remove and insert the cap herself so that you are able to assess her ability to use it safely. When your client has successfully inserted the cap you should re-examine her to check that the cap is fitted correctly (see Figs 4.11 and 4.12).

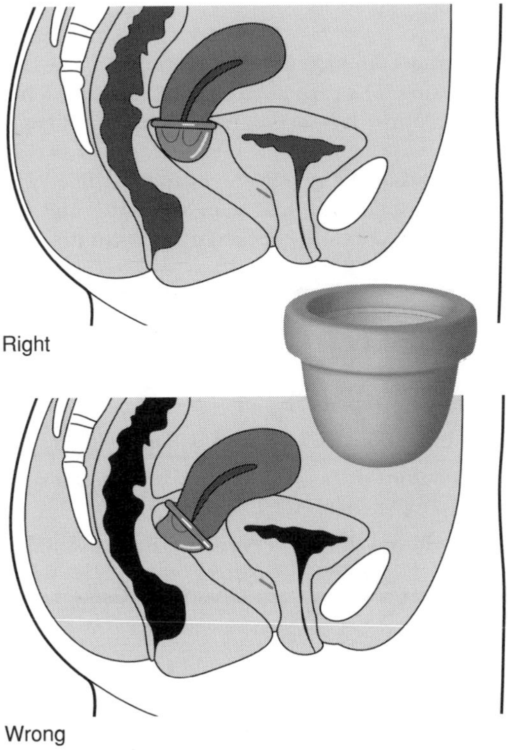

4: Female barrier methods

Right

Wrong

Fig. 4.11 The cervical cap in position. (Reproduced from *Women's Sexual Health*, G. Andrews (ed.), 1996, Baillière Tindall.)

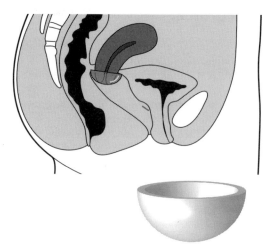

Fig. 4.12 The Dumas (or vault) cap in position. (Reproduced from *Women's Sexual Health*, G. Andrews (ed.), 1996, Baillière Tindall.)

Use of the cap

All caps should be used in conjunction with a spermicide. The cap should be filled by a third with spermicide. The cap should be left *in situ* for 6 hours after the last episode of sexual intercourse. It is recommended that the client inserts additional spermicide into the vagina prior to sexual intercourse. This can either be performed by using a spermicidal pessary or by using an introducer filled with spermicide.

The cap should be washed with mild soap and water and stored carefully. It should be renewed once a year and checked every 6 months.

SELF ASSESSMENT QUESTIONS

Answers and discussion at the end of the chapter.

4. Which preparations do you think will affect the cap?
5. Which situations do you think the client should return early for her cap to be checked?
6. For whom do you think a cervical cap is most suitable?

The future

Research is currently being undertaken on new modified cervical caps. Clinical trials into a custom fitted valved cervical cap known as the contracap showed a high failure rate but it was highly acceptable to women; however, this method had the advantage of not requiring the use of spermicide (Bounds *et al.*, 1986).

Case History

A 30-year-old woman who had previously been fitted with the diaphragm attended complaining that it seemed to be causing increased cystitis. She had ensured that prior to and following sexual intercourse she emptied her bladder, with no improvement.

A Dumas cap was suitable for her and she was taught how to fit this. A follow-up appointment was organized to assess the client's ability to fit the Dumas and see if the bladder irritation was reduced.

A new cervical cap has been launched onto the American market called Lea's Shield which is available in one size and can be left *in situ* for 48 hours. However, as yet there is no research available as to its efficacy.

Sexuality and anxieties

Women who use the cervical cap have often previously used a diaphragm, which ensures that they feel comfortable with their body and have experience of locating their cervix. If a partner has been taught how to fit the cap then this can be incorporated into foreplay. It may also help to give a greater understanding to the relationship.

Many young women attend consultations requesting the 'new cap' thinking the cap is a new innovation. However, a cap may not be appropriate for them and a diaphragm may be more suitable. Like the diaphragm, the cap gives women power over their bodies. It also helps educate women and their partners about the female reproductive system.

THE SPONGE

The sponge was available over the counter but is no longer being manufactured because of a change in production requirements in the USA. The sponge was marketed as the 'Today' sponge.

The sponge was made of polyurethane and impregnated with spermicide. The sponge was designed to be inserted into the vagina with the indented surface covering the cervix. A loop on the other side was provided to aid removal. The sponge was moistened prior to insertion to activate the spermicide. The sponge could only be used for one episode of sexual intercourse.

THE FEMALE CONDOM

Introduction and history

Women have inserted a wide variety of objects into their vagina, from lemons to oiled silk, in order to control their fertility. Femidom is the only female condom available on the UK market. It is available over the counter to all women and has helped to increase the choice open to women.

Explanation of the method

The female condom is made of lubricated polyurethane. It is 170 mm in length and has an outer ring and an inner ring. The inner ring, which is situated at the closed end of the condom, is used to aid insertion. The outer ring is situated at the open end of the condom and lies flat against the vulva. The female condom prevents sperm from entering the vagina by acting as a barrier.

Efficacy

The female condom is similar to the male condom in its effectiveness in preventing pregnancy. There have only been a few studies researching the efficacy of the female condom, but these indicate that the efficacy is similar to that of the male condom – from 85% for typical use to 98% for perfect use (Trussell *et al.*, 1994).

Disadvantages

❖ Perceived as noisy

❖ Requires motivation

❖ May be perceived as interrupting sexual intercourse.

Advantages

❖ Under the control of the woman

❖ Protects against sexually transmitted diseases and HIV

❖ Can be used in conjunction with oil-based products

❖ No systemic side effects.

Contraindications

❖ Present vaginal, cervical or pelvic infection should be investigated and treated first

❖ Inability by client to touch genital area.

Range of method

There is one female condom available in the UK marketed under the name Femidom.

How to teach the use of the female condom

You should advise your client to insert the female condom by squeezing the smaller ring at the closed end of the condom between her thumb and index finger. She should then insert the ring into the vagina as far as she can and insert her finger into the condom. This will push the condom upwards into the vagina, and allow the outer ring to lie flat against the vulva. The inner ring does not need to lie over the cervix, and should be left *in situ* (see Fig. 4.13).

The woman's partner should insert his penis into the condom, with the outer

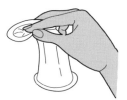
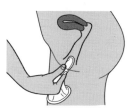

1. The small ring which lies within the closed end of the condom helps to insert Femidom much like a tampon and holds the condom in place in the vagina. To insert, firmly hold the small ring between the thumb and middle finger.

2. Find a comfortable position; either lying down, sitting with the knees apart, or standing with one foot up on a chair. Insert the squeezed ring into the vagina pushing it inside as far as possible.

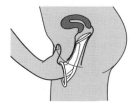
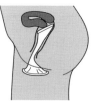

3. Put a finger inside the condom and push the small ring inside as far as it can go, like a tampon. Most women do not feel the inner ring once Femidom is inserted. Some may find that insertion is fully completed by the penis when it enters the vagina. There is no need for Femidom to be fitted over the cervix.

4. It is normal for part of the condom to hang outside the body. The outer ring helps keep the condom in place and will lie flat against the body when the penis is inside the condom. Most couples do not feel the outer ring during use.

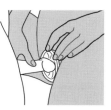
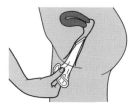

5. The penis should be guided inside the condom. As long as the penis remains inside the sheath and the outer ring remains outside the body, then Femidom is working.

6. To remove, twist the outer ring to contain the semen and gently pull Femidom out. Femidom must be removed before risk of spilling any ejaculate, immediately after loss of erection.

Like male condoms, Femidom can only be used once, and must not be flushed down the toilet.

Fig. 4.13 Step by step guide to using Femidom. (Reproduced with kind permission of Femidom Advice Bureau, Chartex International Plc.)

ring lying flat against the vulva. Care should be taken that the penis is not inserted between the condom and the vagina. Once ejaculation has taken place the outer ring should be twisted so that the ejaculate is retained in the female condom, and gently pulled out of the vagina. The female condom should be disposed of in a rubbish bin; it cannot be flushed down a toilet.

All teaching should be supported by relevant written information.

Counselling

The female condom is suitable for women with a latex allergy. It is also ideal for women who are concerned about HIV and sexually transmitted diseases. It feels stronger and more durable than a male condom and is not affected by oil-based lubricants.

Women can insert the female condom prior to sexual intercourse. They will find that it will stay *in situ* if they move around as long as they have fitted it correctly. Some women have mistakenly removed the inner ring of the condom which helps keep the condom in position.

Although research (Bounds *et al.*, 1992a) has shown that the female condom is not aesthetically pleasing to many women and their partners, a number of positive features were highlighted. These included that the Femidom rarely split, and that there was less loss of sensitivity experienced by men compared with the male condom.

Problems encountered

❖ *PENIS INSERTED OUTSIDE THE FEMALE CONDOM:*
   Clients should be advised to insert the penis carefully and be aware of this problem and informed about emergency contraception.

❖ *FEMALE CONDOM REMOVED AS THE PENIS IS WITHDRAWN:*
   Clients should be encouraged to hold onto the outside ring as the penis is withdrawn.

❖ *CLIENT COMPLAINS OF NOISE:*
   Some women have complained about a rustling noise; others however have commented that they do not mind the sound. The use of additional spermicide or lubrication may help to reduce this problem but this may make the condom more slippery.

SELF ASSESSMENT QUESTIONS

Answers and discussion at the end of the chapter.

7. What advantages do you think the female condom has that would appeal to a woman?

Sexuality and anxieties

The female condom may seem unappealing to some women because of its appearance or the 'rustling sound' made. However in a relationship that is open and understanding this method may be a very acceptable choice. Research (Bounds *et al.*, 1992a) has shown that a small proportion of couples may prefer this method over the male condom as they found sexual intercourse more enjoyable. Other couples have experienced less loss of sensitivity with the female condom.

In another study where the female condom's acceptability and experience was researched (Ford & Mathie, 1993) clients commented that they liked the 'lack of mess'. Some women encouraged their partners to insert the condom which they found enjoyable. Other women found the insertion of the female condom embarrassing and awkward. It was also noted that, like all methods, men and women found insertion easier with prolonged use.

SPERMICIDES

Introduction and history

Spermicides are usually used with another method of contraception such as the diaphragm and condom. They are applied to certain makes of condoms and were present in the contraceptive sponge.

Explanation of the method

Spermicides inactivate sperm by causing changes in the cell membrane of the spermatozoa.

Efficacy

There is little information on the efficacy of spermicides used on their own. They are believed to be of only a moderate efficacy which is why it is recommended that they are used in conjunction with another form of contraception.

Disadvantages

- ❖ Perceived as messy
- ❖ Local allergic reaction
- ❖ Only of moderate contraceptive efficacy.

Advantages

- ❖ Provides lubrication
- ❖ Easily available
- ❖ May provide protection against sexually transmitted diseases and HIV
- ❖ Can be used in conjunction with the barrier methods of contraception.

Absolute contraindication

❖ Allergic reaction to spermicides

Range of method

Spermicides are available in various forms – creams, foams, gels and pessaries. A selection of spermicides is listed in Table 4.1.

Table 4.1 Spermicides		
Name of product	**Chemical constituent**	**Presentation**
Creams		
Ortho-creme	Nonoxynol 9	70 g cream
Foams		
Delfen with applicator	Nonoxynol 9	20 g aerosol
Gels		
Duragel	Nonoxynol 9	100 g gel
Gynol II	Nonoxynol 9	81 g non-scented jelly
Pessaries		
Double check	Nonoxynol 9	10 pessaries
Ortho-forms	Nonoxynol 9	15 pessaries
Staycept	Nonoxynol 9	10 pessaries

Side effect

❖ Local irritation.

SELF ASSESSMENT QUESTIONS

Answers and discussion at the end of the chapter.

8. Which spermicide would you recommend if a client complained of local irritation?

Counselling

Nonoxynol 9 has been demonstrated in laboratory research to be effective *in vitro* against HIV (Chantler, 1992). However these anti-HIV properties may be modified by use *in vivo* (Chantler, 1992). Concern exists over reports of local trauma caused by Nonoxynol 9 and whether this causes vulnerability to HIV transmission (Bird, 1991). Some small studies have shown no increase in genital irritation in infrequent use of Nonoxynol 9, but an increase in genital irritation if used four times a day (Niruthisard *et al.*, 1991; Roddy *et al.*, 1993). Therefore the use of Nonoxynol 9 in HIV prevention requires further wider research.

The future

Current research is investigating the use as a vaginal spermicide of Chlorhexidine which has shown some exciting properties. Chlorhexidine has been shown to be active against HIV without the membrane disruption associated with Nonoxynol 9 (Chantler, 1992).

ANSWERS TO SELF ASSESSMENT QUESTIONS

1. **Which preparations should not be used with a diaphragm?**
   The following preparations should not be used with a diaphragm as they damage the latex rubber: arachis oil enemas, baby oil, bath oil, body oil, butter, cold cream, cooking oil, cream, cyclogest, ecostatin, fungilin, gyno-daktarin, gyno-pevaryl, hair conditioner, ice cream, lipstick, low-fat spreads, massage oil, monistat, nizoral, nystan cream, nystavescent, orthodienoestrol, orthogynest, pimafucin cream, premarin, skin softener, sultrin, vaseline, witepsol-based suppositories.

2. **How would you help a client who is unable to locate her cervix?**
   If a client is unable to locate her cervix then try getting her to assume a different position to feel her cervix, like squatting or with a foot on a chair. You can ask if she and her partner are willing for her partner to check that her cervix is covered.

3. **For which clients would an arcing diaphragm be appropriate?**
   An arcing diaphragm is suitable for a woman with a posterior cervix, or for someone who is having problems locating her cervix or fitting her diaphragm.

4. **Which preparations do you think will affect the cap?**
   The same preparations will affect the cap that affect the diaphragm: arachis oil enemas, baby oil, bath oil, body oil, butter, cold cream, cooking oil, cream, cyclogest, ecostatin, fungilin, gyno-daktarin, gyno-pevaryl, hair conditioner, ice cream, lipstick, low-fat spreads, massage oil, monistat, nizoral, nystan cream, nystavescent, orthodienoestrol, orthogynest, pimafucin cream, premarin, skin softener, sultrin, vaseline, witepsol-based suppositories.

5. Which situations do you think the client should return early for her cap to be checked?

The client should return early for her cap to be checked if she has a problem with fitting the cap or locating her cervix, if she has become pregnant, or if she has any signs of vaginal, cervical or pelvic infection. The client should return if she has any treatment or surgery to the cervix which may change its shape, e.g. loop diathermy. Lastly if the cap deteriorates then this may be less effective and she should return for a new cap to be fitted.

6. For whom do you think a cervical cap is most suitable?

Women who are most suitable for a cap are able to locate their cervix. If they are unable to do this, perhaps because they are disabled, then their partner may be taught how to fit the cap. If a client has poor vaginal muscle tone then a cervical cap may be more appropriate than a diaphragm. If a woman's partner is able to feel her diaphragm and she is suitable then a cap may be fitted.

7. What advantages do you think the female condom has that would appeal to a woman?

The female condom has many advantages that appeal to women. Women who have anxiety over sexually transmitted diseases and HIV because their partner has sexual intercourse outside the relationship, have commented that they prefer this method because it gives them control over contraception combined with safer sex. The female condom may appeal to women who suffer from recurrences in genital herpes. It also gives a wider choice for prostitutes practising safer sex.

The female condom may appeal to women who are physically disabled as it has no systemic effects and can be inserted by her partner as part of foreplay. Any woman or her partner who has an allergy to latex may find the female condom more suitable as it is made of polyurethane.

8. Which spermicide would you recommend if a client complained of local irritation?

If a client complains of local irritation it may be due to irritation to the chemical constituent Nonoxynol 9. Trying a different spermicide may help. It is important to exclude vaginal infection first as the spermicide may be provoking symptoms of an already present infection.

CONTRACEPTIVE PILLS

- ❖ **Introduction**
- ❖ **The combined contraceptive pill**
- ❖ **The progestogen only pill**

INTRODUCTION

Contraceptive pills include the combined pill which contains the hormones oestrogen and progestogen, and the progestogen only pill which contains the hormone progestogen. These are abbreviated to the COC and POP by professionals, and referred to by women in the case of the combined pill as 'the pill' and to the progestogen pill as the 'mini pill'.

Many women choose hormonal methods as their contraception because they are reliable, yet easily reversible, whilst still being under their control. In the UK contraceptive services including contraceptive pills are free from prescription charges, enabling them to be accessible to all women.

There is a wide range of contraceptive pills and with increasing media attention focusing on this area women have a greater knowledge of the types and makes of pills available. However this knowledge often does not extend to guidelines over missed pills, so these cannot be emphasized too much by health care professionals.

THE COMBINED CONTRACEPTIVE PILL

Introduction and history

The combined pill is today one of the most widely used methods of contraception, but the pills currently used are quite different from the original pills. In the late 1930s Dr Kurzrok showed that the administration of oral oestrogen eased dysmenorrhoea and inhibited ovulation. In 1956 clinical trials began in Puerto Rico on a combined oestrogen and progestogen pill called Enovid; it was approved for use in America in 1957. In 1960 clinical trials began in the UK and in 1961 Conovid E and Anovlar, each containing more than 50 µg of oestrogen, were approved by the Medical Advisory Council of the Family Planning Association.

Explanation of the method

The combined oral contraceptive pill contains the hormones oestrogen and progestogen. It prevents pregnancy by:

❖ Inhibiting ovulation

❖ Making the endometrium unfavourable for implantation

❖ Making the cervical mucus impenetrable to sperm.

Efficacy

With careful use the combined pill is 99% effective in preventing pregnancy; however with less careful use the efficacy may be as low as 93%.

Disadvantages

❖ Needs to be taken regularly, carefully and consistently

❖ No protection against STDs and HIV

❖ Increased risk of circulatory disorders such as hypertension, arterial disease and venous thromboembolism

❖ Increased risk of liver adenoma, cholestatic jaundice, gallstones

❖ Effect of COC on breast cancer (see p. 96)

❖ Unsuitable for smokers over the age of 35.

Advantages

❖ Reliable and easily reversible

❖ Relief of dysmenorrhoea and menorrhagia

❖ Reduces risk of anaemia

❖ Reduces the risk of benign breast disease

❖ Relief of pre-menstrual symptoms

❖ Fewer ectopic pregnancies

❖ Reduction of ovarian cysts

❖ Less pelvic inflammatory disease

❖ Protects against endometrial and ovarian cancer.

Absolute contraindications

❖ Pregnancy

❖ Breast feeding

5: Contraceptive pills

- ❖ Undiagnosed vaginal or uterine bleeding
- ❖ Past or present venous thrombosis
- ❖ Past or present arterial thrombosis
- ❖ Cardiovascular and ischaemic heart disease
- ❖ Lipid disorders
- ❖ Focal and crescendo migraines
- ❖ Cerebral haemorrhage
- ❖ Transient ischaemic attacks
- ❖ Active disease of the liver, e.g. malignancy, history of cholestatic jaundice, impaired liver function tests, gall bladder disease, unexplained jaundice
- ❖ Oestrogen-dependent neoplasms
- ❖ Serious medical conditions which are either related to previous use of the combined pill or affected by sex steroids, e.g. porphyrias, hypertension, pemphigoid gestationis, otosclerotic deafness, systemic lupus erthematosus, Stevens–Johnson syndrome, trophoblastic disease, acute pancreatitis, chorea
- ❖ Four weeks before major surgery or leg surgery
- ❖ Obesity (body mass index (BMI) over 35 kg m^{-2}; see Fig 5.1)
- ❖ Severe diabetes mellitus with complications
- ❖ Smokers over the age of 35
- ❖ Family history of arterial or venous disease in a first degree relative below the age of 45
- ❖ Acute episodes of Crohn's disease and ulcerative colitis.

5: Contraceptive pills

Relative contraindications

- ❖ Sickle cell disease
- ❖ Severe depression
- ❖ Inflammatory bowel disease in remission, e.g. Crohn's disease and ulcerative colitis where prothrombotic changes may occur
- ❖ Diseases where high density lipoprotein (HDL) is reduced, e.g. diabetes, hypertension
- ❖ Splenectomy
- ❖ Diseases whose drug treatment affects the efficacy of the combined pill, e.g. tuberculosis, epilepsy
- ❖ Diabetes mellitus (young, healthy diabetics free of diabetic complications who are non-smokers may be given a low dose combined pill)
- ❖ Obesity (BMI of 30–35 kg m^{-2}; see Fig 5.1).

Weight kg	141	144	147	150	153	156	159	162	165	168	171	174	177	180	183	186	Weight st	lb
40	20	19	19	18	17	16	16	15	15	14	14	13	13	12	12	12	6	4
42	21	20	19	19	18	17	17	16	15	15	14	14	13	13	13	12	6	8
44	22	21	20	20	19	18	17	17	16	16	15	15	14	14	13	13	6	13
46	23	22	21	20	20	19	18	18	17	16	16	15	15	14	14	13	7	4
48	24	23	22	21	21	20	19	18	18	17	16	16	15	15	14	14	7	8
50	25	24	23	22	21	21	20	19	18	18	17	17	16	15	15	14	7	13
52	26	25	24	23	22	21	21	20	19	18	18	17	17	16	16	15	8	3
54	27	26	25	24	23	22	21	21	20	19	18	18	17	17	16	16	8	7
56	28	27	26	25	24	23	22	21	21	20	19	18	18	17	17	16	8	12
58	29	28	27	26	25	24	23	22	21	21	20	19	19	18	17	17	9	2
60	30	29	28	27	26	25	24	23	22	21	21	20	19	19	18	17	9	7
62	31	30	29	28	26	25	25	24	23	22	21	20	20	19	19	18	9	11
64	32	31	30	28	27	26	25	24	24	23	22	21	20	20	19	18	10	1
66	33	32	31	29	28	27	26	25	24	23	23	22	21	20	20	19	10	6
68	34	33	31	30	29	28	27	26	25	24	23	22	22	21	20	20	10	10
70	35	34	32	31	30	29	28	27	26	25	24	23	22	22	21	20	11	0
72	36	35	33	32	31	30	28	27	26	26	25	24	23	22	21	21	11	5
74	37	36	34	33	32	30	29	28	27	26	25	24	24	23	22	21	11	9
76	38	37	35	34	32	31	30	29	28	27	26	25	24	23	23	22	12	0
78	39	38	36	35	33	32	31	30	29	28	27	26	25	24	23	23	12	4
80	40	39	37	36	34	33	32	30	29	28	27	26	26	25	24	23	12	8
82	41	40	38	36	35	34	32	31	30	29	28	27	26	25	24	24	12	13
84	42	41	39	37	36	35	33	32	31	30	29	28	27	26	25	24	13	3
86	43	41	40	38	37	35	34	33	32	30	29	28	27	27	26	25	13	8
88	44	42	41	39	38	36	35	34	32	31	30	29	28	27	26	25	13	12
90	45	43	42	40	38	37	36	34	33	32	31	30	29	28	27	26	14	3
92	46	44	43	41	39	38	36	35	34	33	31	30	29	28	27	27	14	7
94	47	45	44	42	40	39	37	36	35	33	32	31	30	29	28	27	14	11
96	48	46	44	43	41	39	38	37	35	34	33	32	31	30	29	28	15	2
98	49	47	45	44	42	40	39	37	36	35	34	32	31	30	29	28	15	6
100	50	48	46	44	43	41	40	38	37	35	34	33	32	31	30	29	15	11
102	51	49	47	45	44	42	40	39	37	36	35	34	33	31	30	29	16	1
104	52	50	48	46	44	43	41	40	38	37	36	34	33	32	31	30	16	5
106	53	51	49	47	45	44	42	40	39	38	36	35	34	33	32	31	16	10
108	54	52	50	48	46	44	43	41	40	38	37	36	34	33	32	31	17	0
110	55	53	51	49	47	45	44	42	40	39	38	36	35	34	33	32	17	5
112	56	54	52	50	48	46	44	43	41	40	38	37	36	35	33	32	17	9
114	57	55	53	51	49	47	45	43	42	40	39	38	36	35	34	33	18	0
116	58	56	54	52	50	48	46	44	43	41	40	38	37	36	35	34	18	4
118	59	57	55	52	50	48	47	45	43	42	40	39	38	36	35	34	18	8
120	60	58	56	53	51	49	47	46	44	43	41	40	38	37	36	35	18	13
122	61	59	56	54	52	50	48	46	45	43	42	40	39	38	37	35	19	3
124	62	60	57	55	53	51	49	47	46	44	42	41	40	38	37	36	19	8
126	63	61	58	56	54	52	50	48	46	45	43	42	40	39	38	36	19	12
128	64	62	59	57	55	53	51	49	47	45	44	42	41	40	38	37	20	2
130	65	63	60	58	56	53	51	50	48	46	44	43	41	40	39	38	20	7
	4'8"	4'9"	4'10"	4'11"	5'0"	5'2"	5'3"	5'4"	5'5"	5'6"	5'7"	5'9"	5'10"	5'11"	6'0"	6'1"		

Height in feet and inches

Fig. 5.1 Chart of body mass index (BMI). (Reproduced with kind permission of Organon Laboratories Ltd.)

5: Contraceptive pills

Range of method

Drug manufacturers have produced a wide range of combined pills (Table 5.1). There are three types of combined pills:

- ❖ Monophasic pills
- ❖ Biphasic pills
- ❖ Triphasic pills.

Monophasic pills

The most widely used combined pill is a monophasic pill, which means that it contains the same amount of oestrogen and progestogen throughout its 21 days of pills, e.g. Brevinor, Cilest, Eugynon 30, Femodene, Loestrin 20, Loestrin 30, Marvelon, Mercilon, Microgynon, Minulet, Ovranette, Ovysmen, Ovran, Ovran 30, Norinyl-1, Ortho-Novum 1/50.

Biphasic pills

These are 21-day pills which contain the same amount of oestrogen throughout the packet but have pills with two different levels of progestogen in them. These are usually coded in different colours, e.g. Binovum.

Triphasic pills

These are 21-day pills which contain varying amounts of oestrogen (usually two different levels) throughout the packet but have three different levels of progestogen in them, which are colour coded, e.g. Logynon, Synphase, Trinovum, Trinordiol, Tri-minulet, Triadene.

Ed pills

Every day (ED) pills are either monophasic or triphasic but are 28-day pills. Twenty-one of these pills contain oestrogen and progestogen and seven of these pills are inactive pills containing no hormones, e.g. Femodene ED, Logynon ED, Trinovum ED, Microgynon ED.

Tricycling

Tricycling is where three cycles of monophasic pills are taken in a row without a break. The pill-free week is then taken at the end of the 3 months, and this is followed by a further 3 packets of pills. This reduces the number of pill-free weeks a woman has, so if she is complaining of problems in the pill-free week, e.g. headaches, then this can reduce the number of headaches she experiences in a year. However, this is not routine practice and may be prescribed in exceptional situations.

Side effects

- ❖ Nausea
- ❖ Breast tenderness and swelling
- ❖ Breakthrough bleeding

Table 5.1 Combined contraceptive pills

Pill type	Preparation	Manufacturer	Oestrogen (µg)	Progestogen (mg)	
Combined					
Ethinyloestradiol/ *norethisterone type*	Loestrin 20	Parke-Davis	20	1	*norethisterone acetate*
	Loestrin 30	Parke-Davis	30	1.5	*norethisterone acetate*
	Brevinor	Searle	35	0.5	*norethisterone*
	Oysmen	Janssen-Cilag	35	0.5	*norethisterone*
	Norimin	Searle	35	1	*norethisterone*
Ethinyloestradiol/ *levonorgestrel*	Microgynon 30	Schering HC	30	0.15	
	Ovranette	Wyeth	30	0.15	
	Eugynon 30	Schering HC	30	0.25	
	Ovran 30	Wyeth	30	0.25	
	Ovran	Wyeth	50	0.25	
Ethinyloestradiol/ *desogestrel*	Mercilon	Organon	20	0.15	
	Marvelon	Organon	30	0.15	
Ethinyloestradiol/ *gestodene*	Femodene (also ED)	Schering HC	30	0.075	
	Minulet	Wyeth	30	0.075	
Ethinyloestradiol/ *norgestimate*	Cilest	Janssen-Cilag	35	0.25	
Mestranol/ *norethisterone*	Norinyl-1	Searle	50	1	
	Ortho-Novin 1/50	Janssen-Cilag	50	1	

Biphasic & Triphasic

Ethinyloestradiol/ norethisterone					
	BiNovum	Janssen-Cilag	35	0.5	(7 tabs)
			35	1	(14 tabs)
	Synphase	Searle	35	0.5	(7 tabs)
			35	1	(9 tabs)
			35	0.5	(5 tabs)
	TriNovum	Janssen-Cilag	35	0.5	(7 tabs)
			35	0.75	(7 tabs)
			35	1	(7 tabs)
Ethinyloestradiol/ levonorgestrel					
	Logynon (also ED)	Schering HC	30	0.05	(6 tabs)
			40	0.075	(5 tabs)
			30	0.125	(10 tabs)
	Trinordiol	Wyeth	30	0.05	(6 tabs)
			40	0.075	(5 tabs)
			30	0.125	(10 tabs)
Ethinyloestradiol/ gestodene					
	Tri-Minulet	Wyeth	30	0.05	(6 tabs)
			40	0.07	(5 tabs)
			30	0.1	(10 tabs)
	Triadene	Schering HC	30	0.05	(6 tabs)
			40	0.07	(5 tabs)
			30	0.1	(10 tabs)

Reproduced from *MIMS*, February 1997, with kind permission of Haymarket Medical Ltd.

5: Contraceptive pills

❖ Depression

❖ Changes in libido

❖ Contact lenses may become uncomfortable – this is usually associated with hard lenses and high dose pills.

Decision of choice of pill

When commencing the client on the combined pill, the risks along with the benefits should be discussed fully, so that the client is able to fully understand and weigh up the risks and benefits to them.

Venous thromboembolism

There is a wide range of combined pills which may seem confusing when choosing a pill for a woman. The pill scare in October 1995 served to increase this chaos. Although the combined pill can only be prescribed by a doctor, it is important for nurses to understand the complexity of this issue so that they can take part in this procedure. The decision of which pill to prescribe will depend on the woman's medical and family history.

The range of combined pills used today is mainly divided into two groups known as second and third generation pills. Pills in Table 5.2 are second generation pills and contain the progestogen Levonorgestrel, Norethisterone or Ethynodiol, whilst the pills in Table 5.3 contain the progestogen Desogestrel or Gestodene and are known as third generation pills.

Table 5.2 Second generation pills: pills containing Levonogestrel, Norethisterone or Ethynodiol

Binovum	Loestrin 30	Norimin	Ovysmen
Brevinor	Logynon	Norinyl 1	Synphase
Conova 30	Logynon ED	Ovran	Trinordiol
Eugynon 30	Microgynon	Ovran 30	Trinovum
Loestrin 20	Neocon 1/35	Ovranette	

Table 5.3 Third generation pills: pills containing Desogestrel or Gestiodene

Femodene	Marvelon	Minulet	Triminulet
Femodene ED	Mercilon	Triadene	

The pill scare was related to three epidemiological studies (Jick *et al.*, 1995; WHO, 1995; Spitzer *et al.*, 1996) which showed that pills containing the progestogen Levonorgestrel, Norethisterone or Ethynodiol (which is converted to Norethisterone) have an excess risk of venous thromboembolism for women of 1 per 10 000 per year. For women taking pills containing the progestogen gestodene or Desogestrel the excess risk doubles to 2 per 10 000 per year (Department of Health, 1995). This research only relates to combined pills. No woman with a medical history of venous thromboembolism should be prescribed the combined pill; this is an absolute contraindication.

When assessing a woman's suitability for the pill, you should screen women for the following risk factors for venous thromboembolism:

- Family history of venous thromboembolism under the age of 45
- Prominent varicose veins
- Obesity (this is considered if the BMI is over 30 kg m^{-2}; see Fig. 5.1)
- Immobility, e.g. wheelchair bound.

When counselling a woman you should discuss the research and risk factors related to the combined pill. Any woman with any risk factor for a venous thromboembolism should, after discussion with her, either be changed to another method of contraception or changed to a pill with a lower risk of venous thromboembolism, which would be a pill containing the progestogen Levonorgestrel, Norethisterone or Ethynodiol (see Table 5.2), as always a low dose pill should be chosen. For the third generation combined pill containing the progestogen Norgestimate, e.g. Cilest, there is insufficient information as to whether or not there is also an increased risk of venous thromboembolism.

Women with a family history of venous thromboembolism should be considered for screening for genetic susceptibility as they may be carriers of the factor V Leiden mutation and thrombophilias; this will help ascertain if the woman is at risk of a venous thromboembolism. The incidence of the factor V Leiden mutation may range from 20 to 40% in patients with recurrent venous thrombosis (Machin *et al.*, 1995), which is why relevant screening is strongly advised. It is important to find out your employer's policy for screening, and where clients may be referred for this.

The Committee on Safety of Medicines advised that women who are intolerant to the second generation pills but who are free of venous thromboembolism risk factors may, if willing to accept the small increased risk of venous thromboembolism, take the third generation pill. Intolerance may be interpreted as minor side effects such as facial spots, acne or breakthrough bleeding which may be exacerbated by changing to a second generation pill.

Arterial disease

Whilst it is important to assess women for risk factors for venous thromboembolism it is equally important to assess for risk factors for arterial disease. Risk factors for arterial disease are:

- Smoking
- Diabetes mellitus
- Mild to moderate hypertension; the combined pill is contraindicated if the diastolic blood pressure is above 95 mmHg
- Family history of arterial disease under the age of 45
- Obesity (BMI over 30 kg m^{-2}; see Fig. 5.1).

You should discuss the risk factors for arterial disease with your client. If your client has more than one risk factor then the combined pill will be contraindicated, and if she is over 35 and has any risk factors then the COC should be discontinued. If there is any family history of arterial disease you should encourage her to check her fasting lipids. Any family history of arterial disease under the age of 45 with no other risk factors necessitates relevant lipid screening. Combined pills containing the progestogens gestodene, Desogestrel and Norgestimate appear to increase high density lipoprotein (HDL) which may have a slightly more beneficial effect on lipid metabolism (Robinson, 1994) and hopefully coronary heart disease (Gillmer *et al.*, 1996). One study (Lewis *et al.*, 1996) on third generation pills and risk of myocardial infarction concluded that although they had an increased risk of venous thromboembolism this may be balanced with a reduced risk of myocardial infarction, but these results should be treated cautiously, especially with regard to smokers. However at present further epidemiological data needs to be accumulated before the potential protection against coronary heart disease can be fully assessed.

When choosing a suitable combined pill you should inform the woman of the risks so that she is able to make an informed decision. Medical histories should be updated regularly, and all issues discussed should be clearly documented, and backed up with relevant information.

Breast cancer

In June 1996 the Collaboration Group on Hormonal Factors in Breast Cancer published their study of re-analysis of world epidemiological data which related to 54 studies of over 53 000 women with breast cancer.

Their re-analysis showed that there is a small increase in breast cancer risk for women taking the combined pill (Collaborative Group on Hormonal Factors in Breast Cancer, 1996). The risk of breast cancer is when the woman is taking the combined pill, and in the 10 years following cessation there is a small increase in the relative risk of having breast cancer diagnosed. After 10 years following stopping the combined pill there is no increase in breast cancer risk. It was also found that women diagnosed with breast cancer who had used the COC had clinically less advanced cancers which were less likely to have spread beyond the breast compared with those in women who had not used the combined pill.

The cumulative risk of breast cancer in young women is 1 in 500 under the age of 35, increasing to 1 in 100 at the age of 45 to 1 in 12 at the age of 75; this is irrespective of the use of hormonal contraception (Faculty of Family Planning and Reproductive Health Care of the Royal College of Obstetricians and Gynaecologists, 1996).

The risks of breast cancer were not associated with the dose, duration or any type of hormone in the combined pill. The results were the same for all ethnic groups, and for those with family histories of breast cancer and different reproductive histories (Faculty of Family Planning and Reproductive Health Care of the Royal College of Obstetricians and Gynaecologists, 1996). Because breast cancer incidence increases with age, so the cumulative excess risk increases with increasing age for women starting and 10 years after stopping the combined pill.

It is important to discuss the risk of breast cancer with women taking the combined pill so that they are informed of this data, and understand its implications.

How to take the combined pill

The combined 21-day pill should be commenced on the first day of your client's period. When she starts the pill on the first day of her period no additional precautions are required; these instructions are the same for all 21-day pills whether they are monophasic, biphasic or triphasic. If the pill is commenced at any other time in the cycle additional precautions are required for 7 days. You should encourage your client to take her pills at the same time each day. Once 21 days of pills have been taken then she should have a 7-day break where no pills are taken; this is known as the pill-free week. Following the 7-day break she should restart the pill on day 8. Each packet of pills will always be commenced on the same day of the week the first packet is commenced.

Loss of efficacy of the combined pill

The combined pill's effectiveness is reduced by:

- ❖ Missed pills – if your client forgets to take her pill and is more than 12 hours late
- ❖ Vomiting – if your client vomits within 3 hours of taking the pill
- ❖ Severe diarrhoea
- ❖ Drugs which are either enzyme inducers or affect the absorption in the bowel (see Table 5.4).

5: Contraceptive pills

Table 5.4 Drugs which affect the efficacy of the pill. Enzyme-inducing drugs reduce the efficacy of the pill by the induction of liver enzymes, which increase the metabolism of the combined pill. Broad spectrum antibiotics affect the bowel flora and as a result the absorption of the combined pill

Drug type	Drug
Enzyme-inducing drugs	
Anticonvulsants	Barbiturates
	Phenytoin
	Primidone
	Carbamazepine
	Topiramate*
Antitubercle	Rifampicin
Antifungal	Griseofulvin
Diuretic	Spironolactone
Hypnotic	Dichloralphenazone
Tranquillizers	Meprobamate
Broad spectrum antibiotics	Penicillins
	Ampicillin
	Tetracyclines
	Cephalosporins
*Drug and Therapeutics Bulletin (1996a).	

Loss of efficacy through drug interaction
Liver enzyme-inducing drugs

If your client is given an enzyme-inducing drug like Rifampicin on a long-term basis then alternative contraception is recommended, e.g. the injectable Depoprovera given at 10-week intervals or an intrauterine device. Women wishing to continue with the combined pill whilst taking anticonvulsant or barbiturate drugs which affect the efficacy of the COC will need to change to a pill containing a higher concentration of oestrogen – at least 50 µg – and tricycle (this means taking three monophasic packets of pill in a row without a break). The pill-free week may also be decreased to 4 days to increase the efficacy of the pill. If breakthrough bleeding occurs then the oestrogen content of the pill should be increased to 60–100 µg once abnormal pathology has been excluded. It takes 4 weeks for the liver's excretory function to return to normal once liver enzyme drugs have been discontinued. It is advisable to allow 8 weeks following cessation before a lower combined pill is commenced.

Broad spectrum antibiotics
Long-term therapy

If your client is having long-term broad spectrum antibiotic therapy (see Table 5.4), e.g. tetracycline for acne, then the combined pill may be commenced on the first day of the next period with no additional precautions required. However if she is already established on the combined pill and commences on long-term antibiotic therapy or changes antibiotic then she will need to use additional contraceptive precautions for 2 weeks. If this runs into the pill-free week then this should be omitted and the next packet started immediately. If the pill is a triphasic or biphasic pill then on completion of the packet she will need to take the last section of pills which match her present packet and omit the pill-free week.

Short-term therapy

For women who require short-term antibiotic therapy then additional contraception is required whilst the antibiotic is being taken and for 7 days after completing the course of antibiotics. If the pill-free week appears during this time it should be omitted and the next packet commenced immediately if it is a monophasic pill. If the pill is a triphasic or biphasic pill then on completion of the packet the woman will need to take the last section of pills which match her present packet and omit the pill-free week.

Missed pill rules

Many women either forget or are given little information about missed pill rules so it is a good idea to check frequently that your client is up to date with current guidelines and has relevant written information to back this up. The importance of this information is often underestimated by both women and professionals; however as poor compliance will affect the efficacy of the combined pill, it is essential that missed pill rules are covered (Fig. 5.2).

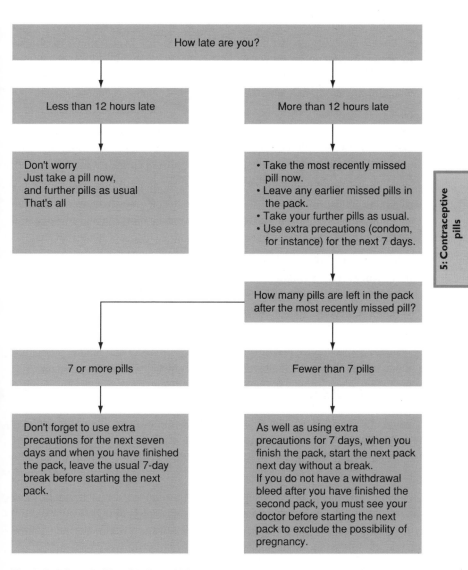

How late are you?

Less than 12 hours late

More than 12 hours late

Don't worry
Just take a pill now,
and further pills as usual
That's all

- Take the most recently missed pill now.
- Leave any earlier missed pills in the pack.
- Take your further pills as usual.
- Use extra precautions (condom, for instance) for the next 7 days.

How many pills are left in the pack after the most recently missed pill?

7 or more pills

Fewer than 7 pills

Don't forget to use extra precautions for the next seven days and when you have finished the pack, leave the usual 7-day break before starting the next pack.

As well as using extra precautions for 7 days, when you finish the pack, start the next pack next day without a break.
If you do not have a withdrawal bleed after you have finished the second pack, you must see your doctor before starting the next pack to exclude the possibility of pregnancy.

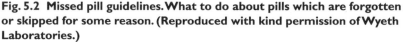

5: Contraceptive pills

Fig. 5.2 Missed pill guidelines. What to do about pills which are forgotten or skipped for some reason. (Reproduced with kind permission of Wyeth Laboratories.)

If your client forgets a pill but it is within 12 hours from when she normally takes it, then she should take it immediately and no additional precautions are required. However if the pill is forgotten more than 12 hours from when it is normally taken then the pill should be taken and additional precautions are required for 7 days of pills. If the pill-free week runs into this time then this should be omitted and the next packet commenced straight away if it is a monphasic pill (see Table 5.1). If the pill is biphasic or triphasic and the pill-free week runs into this time then the pill-free week should be omitted, but the client will need to take enough pills from the end of another packet which match the end of the present packet in colour and dose, and take additional precautions for 7 days following the missed pill. If the pill is an every day (ED) pill and the 7 days of additional precautions required run into the end of the packet, the seven inactive pills should be omitted and the next packet commenced straight away.

If your client vomits within 3 hours of taking the pill or suffers from very severe diarrhoea then the combined pill will not be effective and additional precautions will be required during this time and for a further 7 days once these symptoms have resolved. Again, if this runs into the pill-free week then this should be omitted and if it is a monophasic pill the next packet resumed immediately. If the pill is a biphasic or triphasic pill then your client will need to take enough pills from the end of another packet which match in dose and colour.

Women are safe to have sexual intercourse in the 7-day pill-free week, as long as they do not lengthen this gap. If your client lengthens this gap then she is at risk of ovulating and pregnancy. If she forgets the last pill of her packet she should be advised to count that as the first day of the pill-free week and only have a further 6 pill-free days. If she forgets to restart her next packet on time and has had an 8-day pill-free interval then her pills will not be contraceptively effective until she has taken 7 days of pills; in the meantime she will need to use additional contraceptive precautions. If she is more than one pill late in restarting her packet then emergency contraception may be required.

Initial consultation

Time spent covering the risks and missed pill rules of the combined pill may alleviate future problems and save you and your client time and anxiety in the future. Many women attend having made their contraceptive choice; this does not mean that they do not have absolute contraindications to the combined pill, so a careful medical history of the client and her family is vital. Often a change in contraception is precipitated by unprotected sexual intercourse or an accident with another contraceptive method, so it is important to establish whether emergency contraception is required. Details about the last menstrual period should be obtained as this will help to build a picture of whether there

5: Contraceptive pills

Case History

A 23-year-old woman consults requesting the combined pill. She appears aloof and distant, answering questions with limited replies and poor eye contact. When asked about previous contraception she has recently had 2 years with no contraception, but has been having sexual intercourse. Eventually with time she says 'that things have changed in her relationship' and although she wanted to get pregnant she no longer did. The opportunity to discuss the problems within her relationship are discussed and she decides to see if her partner will attend for couple counselling.

is any possibility of pregnancy. If there has been unprotected sexual intercourse then the client may already be pregnant, and a pregnancy test may need to be performed. Unprotected sexual intercourse is often abbreviated to UPSI.

Look carefully at how your client is sitting, her body language and listen to how she is talking to you and what she is saying. Both men and women can tell you a great deal about themselves from their body language and the feelings they portray.

The risks of the combined pill should be discussed. It is important that your client is aware of the signs of these risks and when to attend early. If your client experiences any of the following problems she should seek medical attention:

- ❖ Pain and swelling in the calf of her leg
- ❖ Chest pain
- ❖ Shortness of breath
- ❖ Increasing headaches
- ❖ Headaches with speech or visual disturbances
- ❖ Pain, tingling or weakness in an arm or leg
- ❖ Jaundice
- ❖ Severe abdominal pain
- ❖ Post-coital bleeding or any prolonged bleeding.

Basic observations should be performed like blood pressure, weight and height. You should calculate your client's BMI, which will help to exclude any absolute contraindications. Details of previous contraception should be covered with any problems your client encountered, as this will help you choose a suitable pill for your client.

Missed pill rules and emergency contraception should be covered, along with when to commence the pill and when efficacy is reduced. Often women do not know how long after unprotected sexual intercourse emergency contraception may be given, and even if they never need to use this information, they may have a friend who does. What is often forgotten is that women learn a great deal from their friends but sometimes this information is inaccurate; on many occasions a client's visit is prompted by a friend.

During your history taking you will eliminate any absolute contraindications to the pill. If there are signs of vaginal infection then appropriate screening should be performed; if this is unavailable then she should be referred to a genito-urinary medicine clinic. If your client is experiencing any post-coital bleeding (often abbreviated to PCB) then she should be referred for a cervical smear along with a bimanual examination. PCB can be a sign of infection, cervical ectopy, polyps or malignancy. If there are no problems then you should record previous cervical cytology and discuss with your client when this needs to be repeated. Women who have not had a cervical smear often fear being forced to have a smear, but if there are no clinical problems then this may be deferred to a convenient time. If your client has any sexual anxieties or problems then she may feel comfortable to discuss them nearer the end of the consultation. Giving time and allowing her to talk will help enable her to approach this difficult subject.

This is a prime time to discuss disease prevention. If your client has a family history of heart disease then it can be useful to discuss blood lipid screening, diet and smoking. You should discuss with your client how the risks of the pill are increased by smoking; if she ceases smoking then these risks will reduce to the same of a non-smoker. It is also a good opportunity to promote breast awareness, and preconceptual screening such as sickle cell screening and rubella status. Although your client may have no intention at the moment of becoming pregnant this is often a good time to perform screening in case immunization for rubella is required.

Women often underestimate the need for protection against sexually transmitted diseases and HIV. There is a belief among many men and women that 'it won't happen to me', and it is often difficult for a nurse to approach this subject when clients are unable to accept this is an issue. However you will need to discuss safer sex and the use of condoms with your client as the pill offers no protection against STDs and HIV and she may not have considered this subject.

Discuss with your client initial problems she may encounter and how to alleviate these, e.g. breakthrough bleeding and nausea (see section on *Problems encountered*) and when you will need to see her again. It is important to inform your client of any potential side effects as this will help alleviate anxiety. Most side effects normally settle within the first 3 months, so it is always worth continuing with a pill, rather than changing to another pill where the symptoms may be perpetuated. A woman commencing the combined pill should be seen in 3 months time. If there are no problems then she should be seen every 6 months from then onwards.

Lastly everything you have discussed with your client should be backed up with up-to-date written information. Often men and women do not read leaflets so you cannot rely on just giving the leaflets – you need to say it verbally as well. It is also possible that your client is unable to read, but may not be prepared to admit this, or that the English language is not her first language. If this is the case try to obtain leaflets in her first language. You should also give telephone numbers where clients can obtain advice and emergency contraception.

The points to be covered at initial consultation are summarized in Box 5.1.

Subsequent visits

At subsequent visits it is important to ascertain whether your client has had any problems of any kind, which may include increasing headaches or migraines. This may be performed by asking open-ended questions like 'how have you got on with your pill?' Allow her time to answer questions. Often clients report that they have no problems, but just as they are about to leave mention that they have had visual problems with a headache or forgotten a pill or not used extra precautions.

Routine observations of weight and blood pressure should be performed. Information about the last menstrual period will help eliminate any risk of pregnancy and also checks that she is taking her pills correctly. Is your client's cervical smear up to date, is she experiencing any problems with her periods or sexual intercourse? Is your client aware of missed pill rules and emergency contraception, does she have up-to-date information? Does she have any anxieties or questions?

BOX 5.1
POINTS TO BE COVERED AT INITIAL CONSULTATION

❖ Full medical history

❖ Family medical history

❖ Basic observations – BP, weight, height, BMI

❖ Has the client had unprotected sexual intercourse and is she in need of emergency contraception or already pregnant?

❖ Cervical cytology and breast awareness

❖ Risks of the combined pill, and when to seek medical attention

❖ Missed pill rules

❖ Emergency contraception

❖ Safer sex

❖ Leaflets on the COC and emergency contraception given to client

❖ Relevant telephone numbers for advice.

If your client has no problems then a prescription for 6 months' supply may be given. It is a good idea to encourage your client to return in 5 months' time so that she has a spare (emergency) packet of pills. Does she need a supply of condoms, is she aware of how to apply a condom or does she need to be taught? If your client is a non-smoker and has no contraindications or complications then she may continue to take the pill until she is peri-menopausal.

The points to be covered at subsequent visits are summarized in Box 5.2.

BOX 5.2
POINTS TO BE COVERED AT SUBSEQUENT VISITS

❖ Update of medical and family history

❖ Basic observation – BP, weight, height

❖ Date of last menstrual period, has she had any problems with her pill?

❖ Is her cervical smear due?

❖ Is she breast aware?

❖ Do missed pill rules need revision?

❖ Safer sex – is she at risk?

❖ Has she got up-to-date leaflets on the COC and emergency contraception?

❖ Have relevant telephone numbers for advice been given?

ACTIVITY

Do you know where your clients can obtain contraception and emergency contraception in your area when you are not working?

Reasons for breakthrough bleeding (BTB) with the COC

It is not unusual for women to have breakthrough bleeding (BTB) in the first 2 months of starting a combined pill; this can be alarming for women if they are not warned beforehand of this possibility. It is important that women continue to take their pill as the bleeding usually stops after two–three packets, and providing all the pills have been taken correctly contraceptive efficacy will not be affected. If bleeding continues beyond three packets of pills then the cause should be investigated, which may be due to:

- ❖ Missed pills
- ❖ Diarrhoea or vomiting
- ❖ Drugs which interact with the COC and affect the efficacy, e.g. enzyme-inducing drugs
- ❖ Disease of the cervix, e.g. cervical cancer, chlamydia
- ❖ Pregnancy
- ❖ Diet, e.g. vegetarians
- ❖ The dose of the pill may not suit the client.

When excluding all possible causes of BTB it is vital to take a detailed history from the woman. This will help ascertain what the cause is and whether contraceptive efficacy has been reduced and emergency contraception is indicated. The type of pill preparation should not be changed until all causes have been excluded. If the BTB is caused by the dose of pill preparation then a pill with a different or higher dose of progestogen should be prescribed.

Problems encountered on the pill

- ❖ *BREAKTHROUGH BLEEDING:*
  Breakthrough bleeding may be due to disease of the cervix, such as cervical neoplasia or chlamydia, so appropriate screening may need to be performed. Pregnancy may cause breakthrough bleeding so this may need to be excluded. If your client has missed pills, had diarrhoea or vomiting then there may be loss of effectiveness of the pill and bleeding. Drugs which cause loss of efficacy of the pill may cause BTB (see Table 5.4). The client may need to change to alternative contraception or change to a higher oestrogen content pill. Women who are vegetarians occasionally have BTB as their enterohepatic circulation may be affected by their bowel flora. Occasionally women who have had extensive bowel surgery may suffer BTB because the absorption of the pill is impaired.
  Breakthrough bleeding may occur because your client has not been on the pill for a long enough duration. It is not unusual to experience BTB in the first few months of taking the pill; this usually disappears so it is important to continue with the pill. However if bleeding is experienced and she has taken the pill for three–four packets with no improvement, and all other causes of BTB have been excluded, then the dosage or type of pill may need to changed. The pill may be changed as the dose of it may be too low; this can be done by choosing a pill with a higher oestrogen content or one with a different progestogen component. It may be necessary to prescribe a pill containing 50 µg of oestrogen.

❖ *YOUR CLIENT FORGETS TO TAKE HER PILL:*

> *It is useful to discuss with your client why she thinks she forgets her pills; this may be because of problems in a relationship, or she may subconsciously desire a pregnancy. If she forgets her pill it can be a useful reminder to keep the pill by her alarm clock, or by the coffee or tea jar, or by her toothbrush. It is a good idea to suggest she carries a spare packet of the pill in her purse so if she has forgotten to take her pill she is likely to have the packet with her. Alarm watches and personal filofax computers can be set to act as a reminder.*

❖ *COMPLAINTS OF NAUSEA:*

> *If your client complains of nausea she should make sure that the pill is taken after eating. If this continues she may need to change to different type of pill or one containing less oestrogen.*

❖ *BREAST TENDERNESS:*

> *If this is experienced in the first 3 months then usually the symptoms resolve. However if your client complains of breast tenderness her breasts should be examined. Evening primrose oil and vitamin B6 can help relieve symptoms if taken continuously. If symptoms persist it may be necessary to change to a pill containing lower levels of oestrogen and progestogen or a different type of progestogen.*

❖ *INCREASED SPOTS AND ACNE:*

> *Try changing to a pill with a different progestogen.*

❖ *WEIGHT GAIN:*

> *Often clients complain of increased weight. Initially they may have a small weight gain, but usually weight gain is due to changes in diet and exercise.*

❖ *VAGINAL DRYNESS AND LOSS OF LIBIDO:*

> *Try to discuss with her any anxieties or problems she may have in the relationship which may be causing this problem. Try changing to a different pill.*

❖ *HEADACHES PRIOR TO PERIODS:*

> *It is important to check that these headaches do not cause focal disturbances as this would be an absolute contraindication to the pill. It may be useful for your client to keep a diary of her headaches and when they occur. If they occur in the pill-free week then tricycling will reduce the number of headaches. Headaches in the pill-free week are usually because the hormone levels have dropped.*

Sexuality and anxieties

The combined pill has given women a greater freedom over their bodies and fertility. The pill has allowed women to choose when they wish to become pregnant.

5: Contraceptive pills

5: Contraceptive pills

SELF ASSESSMENT QUESTIONS

Answers and discussion at the end of the chapter.

1. In what situations would extra precautions be required with the combined pill?
2. Name four beneficial effects the combined pill has on a woman's body'.
3. What are the main concerns or myths about the combined pill that women worry about and how would you answer their questions?

However this has drawbacks – women often find the decision to stop the pill and try to conceive a dilemma. They hope to find the perfect time to become pregnant which will probably never happen, at the same time they feel that time is running out as their body clock ticks ominously away! For some women the pill is too effective; they would like to become pregnant and not have to make the decision.

Women who frequently forget to take their pill may have a subconscious desire to become pregnant, but it may be difficult for them to admit this feeling. Some women have been brought up to believe that sexual intercourse is only for procreation and by taking the pill they are preventing pregnancy, resulting in loss of enjoyment of sexual intercourse.

Women may blame the combined pill for problems which are unrelated to it. Frequent changes of type of pill may indicate an underlying problem. Given time and an empathetic approach these may be vocalized.

Some women feel an enormous amount of guilt for enjoying sexual intercourse with the protection of the pill, and this guilt is often expressed by women who feel that the pill will make them infertile. They feel that there is some divine retribution for being on the pill, and this has been compounded by pill scares. Recently women and their partners have had to read and listen to alarmist articles and news reports in the UK about the pill; the anxiety this has engendered has been enormous. Articles entitled 'the pill can kill' have meant that many women now have a negative image of the combined pill which does not reflect the true properties of it. Women are often surprised at how small the risk of venous thromboembolism and breast cancer actually is! There is also the belief that there should be no risk attached to the pill. This unrealistic view fails to acknowledge the risks of pregnancy, and also the everyday risks we all automatically accept like driving a car or smoking. It is therefore important that we educate and inform women about the risks of the combined pill, and are able to confront the anxieties and alarm they have in a calm and responsible manner (Editorial, 1996). It will take some time before men and women feel as confident about the pill as they did prior to the pill scare.

THE PROGESTOGEN ONLY PILL

Introduction and history

The progestogen only pill used to be referred to as the 'mini pill', which tends to give women the impression that it is of a low contraceptive efficacy. The first progestogen pill was chlormadinone acetate, which was used in 1969 but withdrawn in 1970. There are six progestogen pills (Table 5.5) which have many advantages over other methods that are often underestimated.

Explanation of the method

The progestogen pill (POP) prevents pregnancy in a number of ways. It causes the cervical mucus to thicken, hindering sperm penetrability, and in some cycles it suppresses ovulation; it also renders the endometrium unreceptive for implantation and reduces fallopian tube function.

Efficacy

The effectiveness of the POP is between 96 and 99% in preventing pregnancy. If used consistently and correctly the efficacy will be higher, but for typical use the efficacy will be lower; this may be due to women not taking their pills on time (referred to as user error). Research has shown (Vessey *et al.*, 1985, 1990) that if a woman is heavier than 70 kg there is a trend that indicates that the failure rate is higher, however the numbers were too small in this study to be conclusive. Until more data is available women over 70 kg should be counselled about the possible reduced efficacy of the POP and may be advised to take two progestogen pills a day to ensure contraceptive effectiveness is maintained (Guillebaud, 1993). There is no research at present on efficacy and effects of women taking more than one progestogen pill a day. Much of the research with the POP has failed to differentiate between older women and breast feeding women whose fertility is reduced. This lack of differentiation combined with small studies makes it difficult to give more accurate efficacy rates (McCann & Potter, 1994). However for women who are breast feeding or who are older, e.g. 40 years old, the POP will not only be very suitable for them as a method but also very effective against pregnancy, because of their reduced fertility. One study (Vessey *et al.*, 1985) found that for women aged 40 or more the pregnancy rate was 0.3 per 100 woman years, whilst for women who were aged 25–29 the pregnancy rate was 3.1 per 100 woman years.

Advantages

- Does not inhibit lactation so suitable for breast feeding mothers
- No evidence of increased risk of cardiovascular disease
- No evidence of increased risk of venous thromboembolism
- No evidence of increased risk of hypertension
- Does not need to be stopped prior to surgery

5: Contraceptive pills

Table 5.5 Progestogen only pills

Pill type	Preparation	Manufacturer	Oestrogen (µg)	Progestogen (mg)	
Norethisterone type	Micronor	Janssen-Cilag	—	0.35	norethisterone
	Noriday	Searle	—	0.35	norethisterone
	Femulen	Searle	—	0.5	ethynodiol diacetate*
Levonorgestrel	Microval	Wyeth	—	0.03	
	Norgeston	Schering HC	—	0.03	
	Neogest	Schering HC	—	0.075	norgestrel

*Converted (>90%) to norethisterone as the active metabolite

Reproduced from *MIMS*, February 1997, with kind permission of Haymarket Medical Ltd.

- ❖ Suitable for women with diabetes or focal migraines
- ❖ Reduction in dysmenorrhoea
- ❖ May relieve pre-menstrual symptoms
- ❖ Suitable for women unable to take oestrogen.

Disadvantages

- ❖ To be effective needs to be taken carefully
- ❖ Irregular menstrual cycle
- ❖ A small number of women develop functional ovarian cysts
- ❖ If POP fails may have possible increased ectopic pregnancy rate
- ❖ Effect of POP on breast cancer (see page 110).

Absolute contraindications

- ❖ Pregnancy
- ❖ Undiagnosed genital tract bleeding
- ❖ Past or present severe arterial disease
- ❖ Severe lipid abnormalities
- ❖ Recent trophoblastic disease
- ❖ Serious side effects occurring on the COC which are not due to oestrogen
- ❖ Previous ectopic pregnancy
- ❖ Present liver disease, liver adenoma or cancer.

Relative contraindications

- ❖ Chronic systemic disease
- ❖ Drugs which interfere with the efficacy of the POP, e.g. enzyme-inducing drugs
- ❖ Risk factors for arterial disease (lipid abnormalities may be worsened by POP)
- ❖ Recurrent cholestatic jaundice
- ❖ Sex steroid dependent cancer, e.g. breast cancer
- ❖ Functional ovarian cysts which have required hospitalization.

Range of method

The progestogen only pill contains the same amount of progestogen throughout the packet and is taken every day. Of the six progestogen pills three are made of or convert to the progestogen Norethisterone, and three are made of or convert to the progestogen Levonorgestrel (Table 5.5).

5: Contraceptive pills

Decision of choice

No research has differentiated between different types of progestogen only pills in relation to efficacy, so the choice of progestogen is the one that gives your client fewer side effects and less irregular bleeding. However Microval and Norgeston are the most suitable for women breast feeding as only tiny amounts of progestogen is found in breast milk with these pills (Guillebaud, 1993).

With all progestogen methods the CSAC advises (CSAC, 1993a) that following 5 years of amenorrhoea caused by the POP a serum oestradiol should be taken. If the serum oestradiol is less than 100 pmol l^{-1} then this indicates oestrogen deficiency; additional oestrogen would be appropriate and another method of contraception may be more suitable. Bone density screening may be indicated along with close supervision of the situation.

Research on lipid metabolism and the POP shows that there is a negligible effect (McCann & Potter, 1994). However there may be a decrease in HDL and HDL2 cholesterol. Progestogen pills may be appropriate for women with lipid abnormalities, but this will depend on the severity and close monitoring will need to be performed.

The 1996 Collaborative Group on hormonal factors in breast cancer (Collaborative Group, 1996) found that the risk of breast cancer was similar to that of the combined pill (see page 96).

Side effects

- ❖ Functional ovarian cysts
- ❖ Breast tenderness
- ❖ Bloatedness
- ❖ Depression
- ❖ Fluctuations in weight
- ❖ Nausea
- ❖ Irregular bleeding
- ❖ Amenorrhoea.

How to take the POP

The progestogen pill should be commenced on the first day of a woman's menstrual period with no extra precautions required. The POP is taken every day with no break. If your client needs to change to another progestogen pill then the first pill of the new packet should be commenced the next day with no break and no additional contraception will be required. Broad spectrum antibiotics do not reduce the efficacy of the POP so no extra precautions are required whilst taking them.

If the progestogen only is commenced following a full term pregnancy then it should be started from day 21 after birth; no additional precautions are required. If your client has had a miscarriage or termination of pregnancy then the POP should be commenced the same day or next day with no additional precautions required.

Loss of efficacy through drug interaction

Enzyme-inducing drugs (see Table 5.6) reduce the efficacy of the POP so another form of contraception should be discussed, e.g. the Depoprovera injectable given at intervals of 10 weeks is preferable. If this is unsuitable then she may be prescribed an increased dose of progestogen to three–four pills a day. The efficacy of this regime is unknown and this would be given on a named patient basis after careful counselling.

Table 5.6 Enzyme-inducing drugs which affect the efficacy of the POP

Drug type	Drug
Anticonvulsants	Barbiturates
	Phenytoin
	Primidone
	Carbamazepine
	Topiramate
Antitubercle	Rifampicin
Antifungal	Griseofulvin
Diuretic	Spironolactone
Hypnotic	Dichloralphenazone
Tranquillizer	Meprobamate

Missed pill rules

If your client takes her progestogen pill 3 or more hours late then she should be advised to take her pill when she remembers and use additional contraceptive precautions for the next 7 days of her pill. If a woman has severe diarrhoea or vomits within 3 hours of taking her pill and fails to take another she will need to use extra precautions whilst having diarrhoea and vomiting and for 7 days afterwards.

Initial consultation

When counselling a client initially about the progestogen only pill it is important to explain how this method prevents pregnancy and discuss its efficacy; this will help her to understand why it is necessary to take this type of pill on time. A full past and present medical history should be taken including a family history. If a client has a family history of heart disease then appropriate screening for lipids should be performed. Routine screening of blood pressure, weight and height will indicate whether a client is 70 kg or more in weight and efficacy should be discussed; she may be advised and prescribed to take two progestogen pills a day. This may be done by using two packets at the same time, taking pills from the corresponding days in both packets. Details about the last menstrual period are important and a pregnancy test may need to be performed to exclude pregnancy.

Initial counselling should cover breast awareness, safer sex and cervical cytology history as well as emergency contraception. If there is any evidence of cervical, uterine or pelvic infection then screening and treatment should be undertaken. If a cervical smear is due then this should be discussed with the client. It may be more appropriate to perform this at the next visit in 3 months' time. The progestogen pill will not protect against sexually transmitted diseases or HIV – this issue should be discussed sensitively with the client. Many clients choose to use condoms or spermicides along with the progestogen pill to increase its efficacy; however sometimes men and women fail to think about safer sex.

You should discuss how to take the progestogen pill and when to use extra precautions. Side effects may be experienced initially and you should warn your client that breast tenderness, bloatedness, depression, fluctuations in weight, nausea and irregular bleeding may be experienced. These usually improve with time, so it is important that she continues with the pill as changing pill may perpetuate the problem. Your client may suffer with irregular bleeding which may improve, but pathology should be excluded first. Screening for infection and cervical cytology should be performed along with a bimanual examination. She may also experience amenorrhoea, which may be due to the POP suppressing ovulation. However if there is any likelihood of pregnancy this should be excluded. Given time your client may wish to discuss sexual anxieties, but sometimes clients leave this to the next visit when they know you better. Always give them the opportunity to bring up the subject by giving open-ended questions like 'is there anything else you want to discuss?'

Up-to-date leaflets should be given so that your client can refer to them in an emergency along with relevant telephone numbers. Initially a woman is prescribed 3 months' supply of the progestogen pill and given an appointment for this time.

The points to be covered at the initial consultation are summarized in Box 5.3.

BOX 5.3
POINTS TO BE COVERED AT INITIAL CONSULTATION

- ❖ Full past and present medical history including family history
- ❖ Record blood pressure, weight, height
- ❖ Details of last menstrual period
- ❖ Discuss efficacy of POP
- ❖ Teach how to take the pill and when to use extra precautions
- ❖ Discuss emergency contraception, safer sex, cervical cytology and breast awareness
- ❖ Discuss side effects
- ❖ Give appropriate leaflets and contact numbers.

Subsequent visits

When a woman initially commences the POP she will return for a follow-up visit in 3 months if there are no problems then she should be seen every 6 months after this. Discuss with her how she feels about the progestogen pill, has she taken it on time? Has she had any problems with her pill and what are they? Is she getting a regular menstrual cycle? If her menstrual cycle has been irregular or she has experienced amenorrhoea is this due to failure to take her pill on time, is there risk of pregnancy? A pregnancy test may need to be performed to exclude this.

Routine observations for blood pressure and weight should be performed. You may find that your client is more relaxed at this visit and may wish to discuss sexual problems or anxieties. This is also a good opportunity to discuss and perform cervical smears if due. You may need to revise how to take the progestogen pill as clients have to take in a great deal of information at initial visits and may forget or be confused about missed pill rules.

If there are no problems then a 6 months' supply of the progestogen pill may be prescribed with a supply of condoms if required.

The points to be covered at subsequent visits are summarized in Box 5.4.

5: Contraceptive pills

BOX 5.4
POINTS TO BE COVERED AT SUBSEQUENT VISITS

❖ Upate of medical and family history
❖ Basic observations – BP, weight, height
❖ Date of last menstrual period, has she had any problems with her pill?
❖ Is her cervical smear due?
❖ Is she breast aware?
❖ Do missed pill rules need revision?
❖ Safer sex – is she at risk?
❖ Has she got up-to-date leaflets on the POP and emergency contraception?
❖ Have relevant telephone numbers for advice been given?

SELF ASSESSMENT QUESTIONS

Answers and discussion at the end of the chapter.

4. What problems would you envisage that a woman may encounter on the POP?
5. How would you solve these problems?
6. Which women are most suitable for the POP?
7. Which women are least suitable for the POP?

Problems encountered

❖ *NO MENSTRUAL PERIOD:*
As long as pregnancy has been excluded then you can reassure your client that her pill is working more effectively and preventing ovulation and periods.

❖ *IRREGULAR BLEEDING:*
Check that your client is taking her pills correctly and not taking them late, which may put her at risk of pregnancy. Ask her to keep a diary of her bleeding pattern, so you can review this at the next visit. She may need to change to a different type of progestogen pill, or a different method.

❖ *COMPLAINTS OF NAUSEA:*
Check that she is not taking her pill on an empty stomach. If the problem continues, change to a different progestogen.

❖ *BREAST TENDERNESS:*
Examine breasts. Taking evening primrose oil can help to ease breast tenderness. Changing to a different progestogen may help.

❖ *PROBLEMS REMEMBERING PILLS:*
If a woman is frequently forgetting to take her pill then this will affect the efficacy of the progestogen pill and put her at risk of pregnancy. Check what time she is taking her pill, is there a more convenient time to take it? Can she set an alarm on her watch or computer diary, what about carrying her packet around with her? Discuss with her how she feels about forgetting her pill. Would another method of contraception be more suitable?

Sexuality and anxieties

The progestogen pill may not always be a woman's first choice of contraception. She may have initially requested the combined pill but has a contraindication to

Case History

A 26-year-old woman consults having been on the combined pill for 1 year. She complains of increased headaches and on discussion she says that she is experiencing visual problems with the headaches. When she reads with her headache she finds that she is unable to see words in the text and has been getting some tingling in her tongue. After discussion with the doctor and client other methods of contraception are discussed and the client decides to try the progestogen pill while she considers other methods. She is now unable to take the combined pill as her headaches are focal migraines and this is an absolute contraindication to this pill, but she may be given the POP.

it. This may affect compliance and increase dissatisfaction with the progestogen pill.

Many women hold the misconception that the progestogen pill is ineffective, because it was called the 'mini pill', which may stop women from choosing it. However it is a safe, reliable and effective method if taken consistently by the client.

Women who fail to take their pill on time may subconsciously wish to become pregnant but may not be ready to admit this to themselves. Given time and sensitive counselling they may feel able to discuss this issue.

ANSWERS TO SELF ASSESSMENT QUESTIONS

1. **In what situations would extra precautions be required with the combined pill?**

   Extra precautions are required when the pill's effectiveness is decreased. This may be due to a pill being taken more than 12 hours late from its normal time. Extra precautions are also required if the woman has severe diarrhoea or vomiting or commences a drug which reduces the efficacy of the pill like an enzyme-inducing drug, e.g. Rifampicin, or a broad spectrum antibiotic, e.g. tetracyclines.

2. **Name four beneficial effects the combined pill has on a woman's body?**

   The combined pill reduces the risk of endometrial and ovarian cancer. It reduces benign breast disease, dysmenorrhoea and menorrhagia and as a result of this reduces the incidence of iron deficiency anaemia. There is less risk of ectopic pregnancies and a reduction of functional ovarian cysts. Psychologically the combined pill gives women assurance against unwanted pregnancy and relief of possible disabling pre-menstrual symptoms.

3. **What are the main concerns or myths about the combined pill that women worry about and how would you answer their questions?**

   One of the major concerns that women wish to discuss about the combined pill which is a myth is that 'the pill makes you infertile'. The pill is completely reversible, and does not cause infertility, however no one knows whether they can become pregnant until they do so. A study on primary infertility and the combined pill (Bagwell *et al.*, 1995) concluded that the COC was associated with a lower incidence of primary infertility.

   Another concern women have is related to the length of time they take the pill, they feel 'you should give your body a rest from the pill'. There is no medical reason to stop the pill.

5: Contraceptive pills

Often when women do stop to have a rest this is when they accidentally become pregnant, causing them great anguish. Many women are concerned that the pill is dangerous. In fact the combined pill is a very safe and effective form of contraception. It is not dangerous unless there is a medical contraindication. Smoking is more of a health risk than taking the pill, which is why smokers cannot have the pill after the age of 35.

4. **What problems would you envisage that a woman may encounter on the POP?**

Women may complain of pre-menstrual-like symptom such as breast tenderness, nausea, irregular bleeding or amenorrhoea. They may find it difficult to remember when to take their pill, and if they have taken the combined pill previously they may dislike the lack of warning of their menstrual cycle.

5. **How would you solve these problems?**

Nausea can be solved by always taking your pill after food. Pre-menstrual-like symptoms may be reduced by trying evening primrose oil and vitamin B6. If there is no improvement then changing to a different POP may help.

Problems with irregular bleeding and amenorrhoea should be discussed. Often if women are fully counselled into how the POP works in preventing pregnancy they are more ready to accept any problems. Check they are taking their pills correctly – do they understand the importance of this in relation to efficacy?

6. **Which women are most suitable for the POP?**

Women who are most suitable to take the POP are those who are breast feeding, who are older. It is also suitable for diabetic women, or for women undergoing surgery, or women who suffer migraines or have had a venous thromboembolism or who smoke – all of whom are unable to take the combined pill. There are in fact very few women who are not suitable for this method!

7. **Which women are least suitable for the POP?**

Women who are less suitable to take the POP are women who are unreliable at taking pills or who find the irregular bleeding a problem. It is not suitable for women who are taking liver enzyme-inducing drugs where there will be loss of efficacy. It is not suitable for women who are pregnant or who have had an ectopic pregnancy, or who have been hospitalized with a functional ovarian cyst.

Any woman who has experienced a problem with the combined pill which may not be related to the oestrogen content of the COC or has had a malignancy of the breast should not be given the POP. Women who have any liver disease, arterial disease, lipid abnormality or cholestatic jaundice have contraindications to the POP. Any abnormal bleeding should be investigated first and pregnancy should be excluded as these are also contraindications.

5: Contraceptive pills

INJECTABLE CONTRACEPTION

Introduction and history

Injectables were initially a result of research following the war, when Dr Junkman found in 1953 that a long-acting injection was created if progestogen and alcohol were combined.

In 1957 research began on the injectable Norigest, now known as Noristerat, which is licensed for short-term use in the UK, i.e. following administration of the rubella vaccine. In 1963 trials commenced on the injectable Depoprovera, which was licensed in the UK for long-term use in 1984 when other methods were not suitable. Since 1990 it has been licensed as a first choice method.

Of the two injectables available Depoprovera is the most widely used. However, many women are still unaware of its existence or are given inaccurate information, hindering its acceptance as a method.

Explanation of the method

Like the progestogen pill, injectables prevent pregnancy in a number of ways. They cause the cervical mucus to thicken, thus stopping sperm penetrability, render the endometrium unreceptive for implantation, and reduce fallopian tube function. However the main function of injectables in preventing pregnancy is suppression of ovulation.

Efficacy

The efficacy of injectables is between 99 and 100% in preventing pregnancy. Injectables are a highly effective form of contraception as user failure rates are reduced. This is because women do not have to remember to take a pill and there is no loss of efficacy caused by diarrhoea and vomiting.

Disadvantages

- ❖ Irregular bleeding or spotting or amenorrhoea
- ❖ Delay in return of fertility of up to a year
- ❖ Depression
- ❖ Weight gain
- ❖ Galactorrhoea
- ❖ Once given cannot be withdrawn

❖ May have an association with osteoporosis with long term use
❖ Effect of injectables on breast cancer (see p. 121).

Advantages

❖ High efficacy
❖ Lasts 8–12 weeks
❖ Reduction in dysmenorrhoea and menorrhagia resulting in less anaemia
❖ Reduction in pre-menstrual symptoms
❖ Less pelvic inflammatory disease
❖ Possible reduction of endometnosis because of thickened cervical mucus
❖ Efficacy not reduced by diarrhoea, vomiting or antibiotics.

Absolute contraindications

❖ Pregnancy
❖ Undiagnosed genital tract bleeding
❖ Past or present severe arterial disease
❖ Severe lipid abnormalities
❖ Recent trophoblastic disease
❖ Serious side effects occurring on the COC which are not due to oestrogen
❖ Present liver disease, liver adenoma or cancer.

Relative contraindications

❖ Chronic systemic disease
❖ Risk factors for arterial disease (lipid abnormalities may be worsened by POP)
❖ Sex steroid dependent cancer, e.g. breast cancer
❖ Severe depression.

Range of method

There are two types of injectables, Depoprovera and Noristerat.

Depoprovera

Depoprovera (abbreviated to DMPA) contains depot medoxyprogesterone acetate and is given in a single 150 mg injection deep intramuscularly every 12 weeks. It is now available in a pre-filled syringe.

Noristerat

Noristerat (abbreviated to NET EN) contains norethisterone oenanthate and is given in a single 200 mg injection intramuscularly every 8 weeks.

Decision of choice

Noristerat is licensed for short-term use only; this means no more than two consecutive injections. Noristerat is usually used as a method following vasectomy or rubella administration where a highly effective method is required for a short period of time.

Depoprovera is licensed for long-term use. It is suitable for most women, particularly those who forget their pills, and for women on the COC taking drugs where there is a loss of efficacy. However, there is a lack of information about long-term amenorrhoea, which is usually a result of this injection, and its implications. In 1991 research (Cundy et al., 1991) suggested that women who are using long-term Depoprovera may be partially oestrogen deficient; this may have an adverse effect on bone density and may give an increased risk of osteoporosis. However Cundy et al. (1994) showed that this effect may be completely reversible once oestrogen levels have returned to normal following cessation of Depoprovera. Prospective research is currently being carried out in the UK looking at this area. The CSAC advises (CSAC, 1993a) that following 5 years of amenorrhoea a serum oestradiol should be taken. If the serum oestradiol is less than 100 pmol l^{-1} this indicates oestrogen deficiency. Additional oestrogen would be appropriate and another method of contraception may be more suitable. Bone density screening may be indicated along with close supervision of the situation.

The risk factors for breast cancer for the injectable were found to be similar to those of the combined pill (see p. 96) (Collaborative Group, 1996).

There is no increased risk of cervical (International Family Planning Perspectives, 1992; WHO, 1992) or ovarian cancer with use of Depoprovera; however there is a protective effect for endometrial cancer (Pisake, 1994).

When counselling women about injectables concerning the risk of osteoporosis and breast cancer much of the research undertaken to date is inconclusive. Hopefully studies currently underway will help to resolve this dilemma.

6: Injectable contraception

Side effects

- ❖ Headaches
- ❖ Bloatedness
- ❖ Depression
- ❖ Weight gain
- ❖ Mood swings
- ❖ Irregular bleeding
- ❖ Amenorrhoea.

How to give injectables

Ideally Depoprovera should be given within the first 5 days of a menstrual period; no additional contraception is required. After this all injections should be given every 12 weeks.

Noristerat should be given on the first day of the menstrual period; no additional contraception required. After this all injections should be given every 8 weeks.

Injections should be given deep intramuscularly into the upper outer quadrant of the buttock. The Depoprovera pre-filled syringe should be shaken well before being given. The Noristerat ampoule should be warmed to body temperature before being given. This will make it easier to draw up as it is mixed with castor oil. Both injection sites should not be massaged after administration of the injectable as this will reduce the efficacy of them.

Following first trimester termination of pregnancy and miscarriage the first injection is usually given within the first 5 days with no extra precautions required. Post partum women should commence their first injectable 5–6 weeks following delivery, as if given earlier there is increased and prolonged menstrual bleeding.

Loss of efficacy through drug interaction

There is no loss of efficacy for broad spectrum antibiotics. For enzyme-inducing drugs the interval of the administration of Depoprovera should be reduced, and given at 10 week intervals (Table 6.1).

Table 6.1 Drugs where the time interval between Depoprovera injections should be shortened

Drug type	Drug
Anticonvulsants	Barbiturates
	Phenytoin
	Primidone
	Carbamazepine
	Topiramate
Antitubercle	Rifampicin
Antifungal	Griseofulvin
Diuretic	Spironolactone
Hypnotic	Dichloralphenazone
Tranquillizer	Meprobamate

SELF ASSESSMENT QUESTIONS

Answers and discussion at the end of the chapter.

1. Who would you consider most suitable for using Depoprovera as a method of contraception?

2. What would you do if a woman was beyond 12 weeks for her next Depoprovera injection?

3. Name five issues that should be covered during counselling for women considering the Depoprovera injection.

Initial consultation

Women who consult who are interested in choosing Depoprovera as a form of contraception should be counselled carefully, as this is a less easily reversed method. Counselling should cover the following areas to enable the woman to make an informed decision:

1. Once injected it cannot be removed. It is important that women accept that once given the injection cannot be withdrawn, so any unwanted side effects they experience, although usually short lived, will continue until the injection expires at 12 weeks.

2. Efficacy and frequency of injections. Counselling should involve efficacy and how frequent injections need to be given. Occasionally women have been under the impression that Depoprovera is given every 3 months. This can be longer than 12 weeks, so it is important to talk about frequency of intervals in weeks. If a client is due a holiday, for example, then her injection can be given earlier.

3. Menstrual disturbances. Women should be warned that they may experience irregular bleeding initially with Depoprovera or amenorrhoea within the first year. If warned beforehand then women usually find this acceptable.

4. Return of fertility. There can be a delay in the return of periods and fertility, however most women will become pregnant within 1 year from stopping Depoprovera. There is no evidence that Depoprovera causes permanent infertility. If a woman is thinking of becoming pregnant in the near future then another form of contraception may be more appropriate.

5. Weight gain and other minor side effects. There may be a small weight gain, so if women are aware of this they will be able to monitor it and it may be avoided.

6. Depression may be experienced by some women, although this may be due to outside factors.

7. Long-term use and the possible risk of osteoporosis are at present being researched. Clients often ask about the long term effects of amenorrhoea, and as new information comes to light they should be informed.

Women may wish to be given time before commencing injectables to think about their decision. Timing of the initial injection should be discussed along with alternative contraception. The first injection should be administered within the first 5 days of the cycle, otherwise contraceptive precautions will be required for 7 days. If there has been any unprotected sexual intercourse or there is any concern over pregnancy then a pregnancy test and bimanual examination if appropriate may need to be performed to exclude pregnancy.

Routine observations of weight, height and blood pressure should be monitored. A full medical of the woman and family history should be obtained. Previous contraceptive history should be discussed. If she has used a progestogen method previously this will give an impression of how she will experience the injectable. A cervical smear may need to be performed if due, although this may

6: Injectable contraception

have to be deferred until the next injection if it is during her menses or if she prefers. Injectables do not protect against sexually transmitted diseases and HIV so issues around safer sex may need to be discussed and approached with the woman.

Up-to-date literature about the injectable should be given, along with an appointment when the next injection will be due.

The points to be covered at the initial consultation are summarized in Box 6.1.

BOX 6.1
POINTS TO BE COVERED AT INITIAL CONSULTATION

❖ Full past and present medical history including family history

❖ Record BP, weight, height

❖ Details of last menstrual period and any unprotected sexual intercourse

❖ Discuss efficacy of injectable

❖ Discuss intervals when injectables should be given

❖ Discuss emergency contraception, safer sex, cervical cytology and breast awareness

❖ Discuss side effects and issues around Depoprovera (nos 1–7)

❖ Give appropriate leaflets and contact numbers.

Subsequent visits

Subsequent injections of Depoprovera should be given every 12 weeks and Noristerat at 8 week intervals. Observations of blood pressure and weight should be performed. Regular weight checks can be useful as often clients complain that their weight has increased, yet when weighed there is no change.

At subsequent consultations it is important to find out how your client is finding her injection. Is she experiencing any problems? How can these be alleviated? (see *Problems encountered*). Most side effects of injectables are short-lived like breakthrough bleeding, so it is worth persevering with this method.

BOX 6.2
POINTS TO BE COVERED AT SUBSEQUENT VISITS

❖ Update of medical and family history

❖ Basic observations – BP, weight

❖ Has she had any problems, e.g. bleeding?

❖ Is her cervical smear due?

❖ Is she breast aware?

❖ Safer sex – is she at risk?

❖ Has she got up-to-date leaflets on the injectable?

❖ Have relevant telephone numbers for advice been given?

It is important that your client knows when her next injection will be due, and keeps a record of the date of her previous injection in case she has to attend another nurse or doctor for her injection.

The points to be covered at subsequent visits are summarized in Box 6.2.

Problems encountered

❖ *IRREGULAR BLEEDING PATTERN:*
If a woman suffers irregular bleeding she should be advised to return back before her next injection is due, so that it can be given earlier. If there is no improvement in the bleeding pattern then she may be prescribed concurrent oestrogen either by the combined pill or if this is contraindicated by giving hormone replacement therapy.

Most women who experience breakthrough bleeding find that this resolves usually by the fourth injection.

❖ *COMPLAINTS OF INCREASED ACNE AND MOOD SWINGS:*
Some women may complain of increased acne or mood swings. This usually improves, but vitamin B6 and evening primrose oil may be beneficial. If there is no improvement in symptoms then this should be discussed with the woman. She may wish to change method or treat the acne for example if she has a limited choice of contraception.

❖ *CLIENTS ATTENDING LATE FOR INJECTIONS:*
Women who regularly attend late for their injections may need help with reminders. Some family planning clinics run domiciliary services for this reason, or send their clients reminders. Try making your client's next appointment earlier at 10–11 week intervals.

If your client is beyond 12 weeks since her last injection of Depoprovera then you may need to give emergency contraception if there has been any unprotected sexual intercourse, and pregnancy should be excluded before the next injection is given. Additional contraception is required for 7 days afterwards.

The future

Research (Mishell, 1994) has been undertaken into monthly injectables. Although they showed improved cycle control, reasons for discontinuation were abnormal bleeding and missed appointments. Cyclofem and Mesigyna, two monthly injectables which contain oestrogen and progestogen, have been widely researched. Studies so far indicate the need for careful counselling to avoid women delaying or missing appointments.

Sexuality and anxieties

Injectables are a highly effective form of contraception. They give a great deal of freedom to a woman, only requiring a consultation every 8–12 weeks. They allow women time to think and delay decisions about permanent methods of contraception. However they are not a widely used method. Many women hold misconceptions about the injectable which may also be held by professionals. Fears that the injection causes permanent infertility and foetal abnormality have been researched (Wilson, 1993). Although no evidence has been found to support these anxieties, they still remain. In the meantime injectables are in many instances undervalued and many women are not even informed of the availability of this method.

Many women feel that having an injection which causes amenorrhoea is unnatural. There is concern about menstrual loss – 'Where does it all go?' 'Doesn't all the blood build up?' – which emphasizes the need to explain clearly how the reproductive cycle works and how it is affected by the injectable. Women often forget that during pregnancy and whilst breast feeding there is little or no bleeding and this is natural. However for some women the experience of amenorrhoea can be too worrying. A period is the way women normally know whether they are pregnant or not, and can be very reassuring.

ANSWERS TO SELF ASSESSMENT QUESTIONS

1. **Who would you consider most suitable for using Depoprovera as a method of contraception?**
   Women who are most suitable for Depoprovera are:

   ❖ Women who do not want to become pregnant but are not yet ready to choose sterilization, or do not wish to become pregnant in the forseeable future

   ❖ Women who are having treatment with liver enzyme-inducing drugs, e.g. Rifampicin for tuberculosis

   ❖ Women who are unable to take the combined pill

   ❖ Young women who want a highly effective form of contraception, but either do not want to take the COC or have an absolute contraindication to it, or find it difficult to remember to take it.

2. **What would you do if a woman was beyond 12 weeks for her next Depoprovera injection?**
   If your client has gone beyond 12 weeks then the need for emergency contraception will need to be assessed. Prior to giving the next injection pregnancy will need to be excluded, and additional contraception used until it is given and for 7 days afterwards.

3. **Name five issues that should be covered during counselling for women considering the Depoprovera injection.**
   Five issues that should be discussed during counselling include:

1. Efficacy
2. Delay in return of fertility
3. Amenorrhorea and irregular bleeding pattern
4. Once given the injection cannot be withdrawn
5. Side effects, e.g. weight gain, depression and long-term effects of injectables which are uncertain like research into osteoporosis.

6: Injectable contraception

CONTRACEPTIVE IMPLANTS

Introduction and history

In 1966 The Population Council commenced research into implants, which showed that silastic rubber capsules released continuous levels of steroid hormone for more than a year. In 1975 the first long-term trial was initiated with six elastomer capsules called Norplant. In May 1993 Norplant was approved for use in the UK as a contraceptive.

Explanation of method

Norplant consists of six capsules, each containing 38 mg of the progestogen levonorgestrel, which are inserted subdermally and provide contraception for 5 years (Fig. 7.1).

Norplant prevents pregnancy by causing the cervical mucus to become thicker and impenetrable to sperm. Research has shown that the average daily dose of 30 µg of levonorgestrel which is released by Norplant causes suppression of

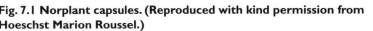

Fig. 7.1 Norplant capsules. (Reproduced with kind permission from Hoeschst Marion Roussel.)

ovulation in 50% of menstrual cycles (The Population Council, 1990). Norplant makes the endometrium unfavourable to implantation, and in cycles where ovulation occurs decreases natural progesterone secretion during the luteal phase.

Efficacy

Norplant is a highly effective form of contraception. Norplant is almost 100% effective in preventing pregnancy. Research (Sivin, 1988; Darney *et al.*, 1990) has shown that in the first and second year there were 0.2 pregnancies per 100 woman years of use. In the third year the pregnancy rate for Norplant was 0.9 per 100 woman years, and for the fourth and fifth years the pregnancy rates were 0.5 and 1.1 per 100 woman years (Darney *et al.* 1990).

Norplant's failure rate is method failure rate rather than compliance failure, which is why it has a high efficacy. Norplant has a high efficacy because it has a no user failure rate – there is no need to remember to take a pill or insert a diaphragm. Studies have shown that for women who weigh more than 70 kg the gross cumulative 5-year pregnancy rate is slightly higher than for lighter women (Sivin, 1988).

Disadvantages

- ❖ Requires trained professional to insert and remove implants
- ❖ Irregular menstrual bleeding for the first year
- ❖ Slight increased risk of ectopic pregnancy
- ❖ Slight increased risk of asymptomatic functional ovarian cysts.

Advantages

- ❖ High efficacy
- ❖ Easily reversed
- ❖ Lasts 5 years
- ❖ Free from oestrogen side effects
- ❖ Low user failure – once in place there is nothing to remember.

Absolute contraindications

- ❖ Pregnancy
- ❖ Undiagnosed genital tract bleeding
- ❖ Allergy to levonorgestrel
- ❖ Present liver disease, benign or malignant liver tumours
- ❖ Sex hormone dependent neoplasms
- ❖ Past or present history of arterial disease
- ❖ Past or present history of thromboembolic disease
- ❖ Risk of ischaemic heart disease, e.g. family history or raised lipid profile
- ❖ Trophoblastic disease.

Relative contraindications

- ❖ Benign breast disease
- ❖ Diabetes
- ❖ Hypertension
- ❖ Migraines
- ❖ Gall bladder, heart or kidney disease
- ❖ Raised lipid profile
- ❖ Severe anaemia
- ❖ Depression
- ❖ History of ectopic pregnancy.

Range of method

Norplant is the only implant available in the UK. It is made up of six flexible closed capsules 34 mm long with a diameter of 2.4 mm made of elastomer. Each capsule contains 38 mg of the progestogen Levonorgestrel.

Side effects

- ❖ Irregular menstrual bleeding
- ❖ Amenorrhoea
- ❖ Pain, itching or infection at insertion site
- ❖ Headaches
- ❖ Nausea
- ❖ Mood changes
- ❖ Dizziness
- ❖ Weight changes
- ❖ Acne
- ❖ Dermatitis
- ❖ Mastalgia
- ❖ Hirtsutism
- ❖ Hair loss
- ❖ Vaginitis.

Decision of choice

Women who are at risk of pregnancy or who have become pregnant because they have difficulty remembering to take a contraceptive pill or use another contraceptive method (user failure) may find Norplant a useful alternative.

Women choosing Norplant as their method of contraception should be counselled carefully about side effects, as this will influence their final decision. If your client has a history of ectopic pregnancy which is a relative contraindication she should be advised that the risk of ectopic pregnancy may increase with duration of Norplant (The Population Council, 1990). However as Norplant is very effective the risk of conception is very low, and as a result the risk of ectopic pregnancy with Norplant is 1.3 per 1000 woman years.

Norplant is suitable for women who have completed their families or for women wishing to delay starting their family. Research has shown that 20% of women wishing to conceive achieved this 1 month following removal of Norplant and a further 50% became pregnant within 3 months (Sivin, 1988), illustrating the reversibility of Norplant.

Counselling for Norplant

As Norplant involves a minor operation it is important to counsel women fully so that they are able to make an informed decision. Women are also more likely to accept and continue with a method if they are aware of any side effects prior to the procedure.

You should discuss with your client the efficacy of Norplant, and the procedure for insertion and removal. A full medical history should be taken along with family medical history. Side effects with Norplant are similar to any progestogen only method, so if your client has previously tolerated a progestogen only method well, then this will give you both a good indication on how she will feel with Norplant. If your client already suffers from symptoms such as headaches or acne then Norplant may not improve these problems. However many women, if warned, are prepared to accept continuing problems to be assured of a highly effective form of contraception.

Changes in menstrual pattern are the most frequently reported side effect of Norplant. Women may experience amenorrhoea, irregular menses or breakthrough bleeding. It is important to discuss the likelihood of amenorrhoea with Norplant as this may cause anxiety. Many women find periods very reassuring as they tell them that they are not pregnant, and as a result amenorrhoea can cause great anxiety. Irregular bleeding is most likely to occur during the first year, but this usually diminishes after 9–12 months of use (Roussel Laboratories Ltd, 1994). Research on clinical experience with Norplant has shown that if women are given careful counselling on Norplant's effects on menstruation there is a higher continuation rate with this method (Mascarenhas et al., 1994).

Following counselling written up-to-date information should be given, so that your client is able to make an informed decision about Norplant.

It is important that your client uses contraception up to the time of Norplant insertion to exclude any possibility of pregnancy. Norplant should be preferably inserted on the first day of your client's menstrual period, where no extra precautions will be required. If Norplant is inserted at any other time in the cycle then pregnancy should be excluded first, and additional contraception should be used following insertion for 7 days.

Following a termination of pregnancy Norplant may be inserted immediately; if inserted later then additional contraception will be required for 7 days. After childbirth Norplant may be inserted on day 21; if inserted later then extra contraceptive precautions will be required for 7 days.

The areas to be covered at counselling are summarized in Box 7.1.

BOX 7.1
AREAS TO BE COVERED AT COUNSELLING

- ❖ Full medical history
- ❖ Check blood pressure, weight and height
- ❖ Ensure client has contraceptive cover up to and after insertion if needed
- ❖ Take details of last menstrual period, exclude pregnancy if relevant
- ❖ Discuss how Norplant works and its efficacy
- ❖ Discuss insertion and removal procedure
- ❖ Discuss side effects
- ❖ Give literature on Norplant
- ❖ Organize date for insertion.

Drugs which reduce the efficacy of Norplant

The drugs which may reduce the efficacy of Norplant are listed in Table 7.1 (Roussel Laboratories Ltd, 1994).

Table 7.1 Drugs which reduce the efficacy of Norplant

Drug type	Drug
Anticonvulsants	Barbiturates
	Carbamazepine
	Phenytoin
	Primidone
Antitubercle	Rifampicin
Antifungal	Griseofulvin
NSAID	Phenylbutazone

Loss of efficacy of Norplant

Additional contraception is required with Norplant whilst drugs that may reduce its efficacy are taken for a short term and for 7 days after they have been ceased. If drugs which reduce the efficacy of Norplant are taken for more than 4 weeks then additional contraception is required for 28 days following their cessation (Roussel Laboratories Ltd, 1994).

Norplant insertion

Norplant is inserted with a sterile technique under local anaesthetic into the inner aspect of the upper arm of the non-dominant arm (Figs. 7.2–7.6). A small

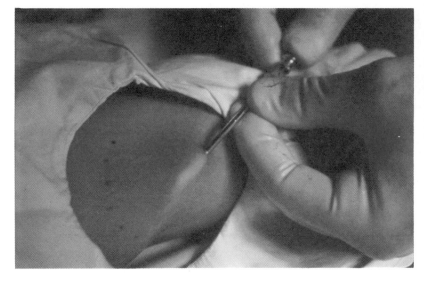

Fig. 7.2 Inserting the trocar under the skin. (Reproduced with kind permission from Hoeschst Marion Roussel.)

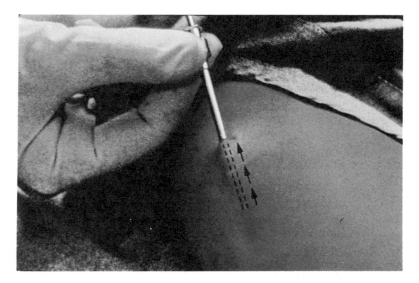

Fig. 7.3 Removing the plunger from the trocar so that the capsule can be inserted into the trocar. (Reproduced with kind permission from Hoeschst Marion Roussel.)

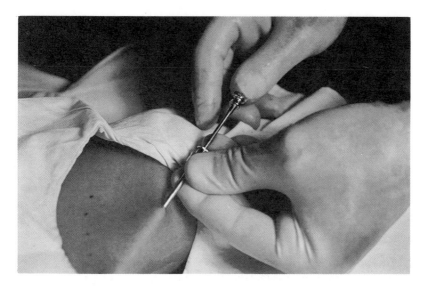

Fig. 7.4 The plunger is reinserted to gently advance the capsule towards the tip of the trocar. The trocar is removed once the capsule is lying beneath the skin. (Reproduced with kind permission from Hoeschst Marion Roussel.)

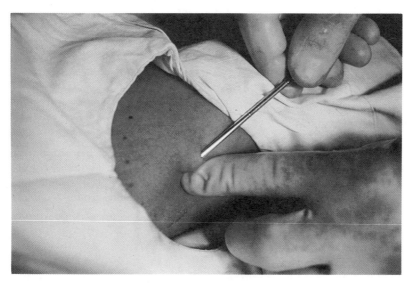

Fig. 7.5 Second capsule being inserted whilst first capsule is fixed in position by finger. (Reproduced with kind permission from Hoeschst Marion Roussel.)

7: Contraceptive implants

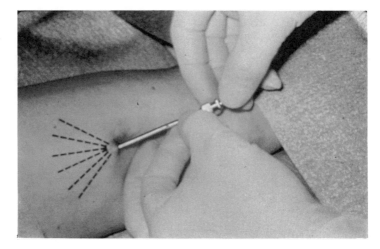

Fig. 7.6 Fan-shaped formation of capsules. (Reproduced with kind permission from Hoeschst Marion Roussel.)

incision is made where the implant capsules are to be inserted via a trocar. The Norplant capsule is inserted under the dermis; the next capsule is inserted 15 degrees from the last capsule. All the capsules should be at a 15 degree angle to form a fan-shaped pattern. Once all the capsules are inserted the trocar is removed, and steri-strips are applied to the incision. A pressure bandage is applied, the steri-strips may be removed in 3 days and the bandage in 24 hours. The insertion procedure takes 15 minutes.

Women should be able to feel the capsules once *in situ* if they wish to touch the site for reassurance, but they will not be visible unless the woman is very thin.

Subsequent visits

You should see your client 3 months after insertion to check her insertion site, blood pressure and weight. If she has no problems then she should be seen at six months intervals for monitoring of menstrual cycle, blood pressure and weight. If your client has menstrual irregularities or pain, or swelling around the implant site then she should be advised to return earlier.

Norplant removal

Removal of the implants is performed under sterile technique with local anaesthetic. The removal procedure takes longer than the insertion procedure. An incision of 4 mm in length is made, and then the capsules are separated from the surrounding tissue by forceps. The proximal end of the capsule is compressed by the doctor (trained in implant insertion and removal) removing the implants, and the other end of the capsule grasped by forceps and gently removed when it becomes visible (Fig. 7.7). This is continued with each capsule until all of them have been removed.

If your client wishes to continue using Norplant as a method of contraception, then a new set of capsules may be inserted in the opposite direction from those removed. However if she is discontinuing with this method alternative contraception is required once the capsules are removed.

7: Contraceptive implants

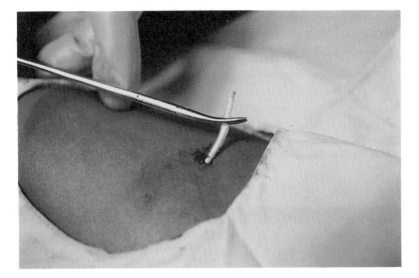

Fig. 7.7 Removal of Norplant capsule. (Reproduced with kind permission from Hoeschst Marion Roussel.)

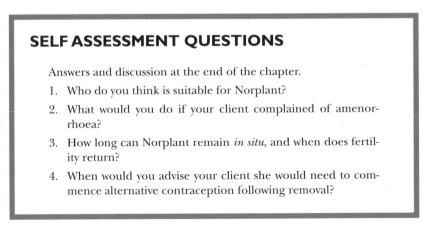

SELF ASSESSMENT QUESTIONS

Answers and discussion at the end of the chapter.

1. Who do you think is suitable for Norplant?

2. What would you do if your client complained of amenorrhoea?

3. How long can Norplant remain *in situ*, and when does fertility return?

4. When would you advise your client she would need to commence alternative contraception following removal?

Problems encountered

❖ *LOCALIZED SKIN REACTIONS:*
 Recent research (Blain et al., 1996) has shown that factors that influence local-ized skin reactions include the use of latex gloves for insertion and removal of the implant, and tension under the first steri-strip applied to the incision.

❖ *IRREGULAR BLEEDING:*
 Research has shown that one of the main reasons for discontinuing with Norplant is due to complaints of irregular bleeding (Diaz et al., 1996); 3.9 per 100 women discontinued because of this problem. This emphasizes the need for comprehensive counselling prior to insertion.

 Women who experience amenorrhoea with Norplant may be alarmed at the loss of their menses if they are not warned prior to insertion. Explaining how Norplant prevents pregnancy and why amenorrhoea occurs can help prevent anxiety.

❖ *PRE-MENSTRUAL LIKE SYMPTOMS:*
 Women may find that taking evening primrose oil or vitamin B6 will help relieve pre-menstrual like symptoms such as irritability and mood swings.

Case History

A 26-year-old woman named Jan has two children aged 2 and 3. She has had a miscarriage prior to having her children, and 3 months ago a ter-mination of pregnancy. Jan has requested a sterilization but her pre-sent relationship is a new one, and it has been suggested that she waits a little longer. She is 5'3" (159 cm) and weighs 15 stone 2 lb (96 kg) and was taking the combined pill but has changed to the progestogen pill, which she finds difficult to remember to take on time. Jan has always suffered from painful, heavy periods and all her pregnancies have been unplanned.

The combined pill is contraindicated in this situation because the BMI is 38 kg m^{-2}. Because of Jan's weight the efficacy of the POP may be affected, and she is unsuitable for an IUCD because of her dysmen-orrhoea and menorrhagia.

On discussion with Jan three long-term methods of contraception are discussed: the injectable Depoprovera, the implant Norplant and the intrauterine system (IUS) Mirena. Jan is reluctant to have the IUS because she does not like the idea of the insertion. She feels that she may not remember to attend for injections every 11–12 weeks, leaving Norplant as the method of choice. Although she is not keen on the insertion of Norplant she prefers this over a Mirena insertion, and decides to go ahead with this as a method of contraception.

The future

At present clinical trials are underway on the acceptability and efficacy of a single contraceptive implant (Coutinho *et al.*, 1996). The single silastic implant contains the progestogen Normegestrol acetate; it is known as Uniplant and provides contraception for 1 year.

Research is also underway on biodegradable implants and other sustained release progestogen implants. One of the complaints with these methods is the occurrence of menstrual irregularities. However single implants would make insertion and removal of the device easier for the woman and the doctor.

Sexuality and anxieties

Women who choose Norplant find its high efficacy and lack of user compliance important advantages. They may be unable to use other methods because of medical contraindications, or wish to use a method that is long term without making the final permanent decision of sterilization.

Norplant has however been beset by problems and misleading information by the media has discouraged uptake by women (*The Economist*, 1995; Bromham, 1996). Problems with removal of Norplant have been widely covered and it has been found that correct placement of the capsules is vital for a problem-free removal procedure. Problems with removal may be because the capsules have been inserted too deeply, making removal difficult. This emphasizes the need to have an appropriately trained professional inserting the implant. The UK distributors of Norplant have established a free training programme for doctors to teach insertion and removal techniques to alleviate this problem. The Faculty of Family Planning have introduced a letter of competence in Subdermal Contraceptive Implants for Faculty members for 5 years from issue and they have developed a regional network of advisors. This has been instigated to validate implant training. Sadly the media influences women and poor publicity about a method remains in their mind. Many forget the risks of pregnancy and childbirth, and the trauma of a termination of pregnancy.

Research has shown (Ruminjo *et al.*, 1996) that of women who used Norplant in two African countries, 90.1% of the 155 5-year users reported a very favourable experience. Other areas of research have shown that many women hold misconceptions about Norplant (Cushman *et al.*, 1996), believing it to be associated with long-term health problems, fertility problems, infection, problems for future babies and expensive. These beliefs were found to be the reason why women failed to choose Norplant as their method. In a smaller study (Fowler, 1996) 47 women were interviewed about their experience with Norplant and the effects of adverse publicity. Forty-four of the women (93.6%) were pleased with Norplant, and all the women felt that it had lived up to their expectations; 11 women had been concerned about media reports. All of the above research emphasizes the need to counsel women carefully about Norplant and discuss the effects of media reports.

The introduction of Norplant has given women a wider choice of contraception, and offers long-term safety against pregnancy. It gives greater freedom to

7: Contraceptive implants

women who have a limited range of methods to choose from because of medical contraindications, yet is easily reversible once removed, but highly effective when *in situ.*

7: Contraceptive implants

ANSWERS TO SELF ASSESSMENT QUESTIONS

1. **Who do you think is suitable for Norplant?**
   Women who are most suitable for Norplant are women who have completed their families, or who do not wish to have children in the near future. Norplant is also suitable for women who may be unable to use another method because they have a contraindication to them, e.g. the combined pill and focal migraines or menorrhagia and the IUCD.

2. **What would you do if your client complained of amenorrhoea?**
   It is important to exclude pregnancy first. Once this has been excluded then you should discuss with your client why amenorrhoea occurs with Norplant.

3. **How long can Norplant remain *in situ*, and when does fertility return?**
   Norplant can remain *in situ* for 5 years. Fertility returns immediately the capsules are removed.

4. **When would you advise your client she would need to commence alternative contraception following removal?**
   Another method of contraception should be used immediately Norplant is removed.

THE INTRAUTERINE DEVICE (IUD)

Introduction and history

It is difficult to find the origin of intrauterine devices. Arabs are believed to have inserted stones into the uteruses of their camels to stop them becoming pregnant whilst on long journeys across the desert. The first IUD in 1909 designed to prevent conception was a ring made of silkworm gut by Dr Richter. In the 1920s Ernst Graefenberg developed a silver ring known as the Graefenberg ring. In many countries contraception was illegal during this time, and antibiotics had not been developed to treat pelvic infection. Later in 1934 Ota in Japan developed the Ota ring, a modification of the Graefenberg ring. In 1962 Dr Lippes introduced an IUD made of plastic called the Lippes Loop. It was not until 1965 that IUDs became available to women through Family Planning Clinics, and in 1969 copper wire was added to the IUD which was found to increase the efficacy of the device. The IUD is often referred to as the 'coil'.

Recently newer IUDs have been introduced which have fewer side effects, increased efficacy and last up to 10 years. With the commencement of chlamydia screening IUDs have been given a new lease of life. The development of the intrauterine system Mirena, a progestogen-releasing intrauterine device, has meant that the choice of contraception has now widened.

Explanation of method

An intrauterine device is inserted through the cervical canal and sits in the uterus. It has threads which hang down into the vagina, which a woman can check to make sure that the device is correctly positioned. It prevents pregnancy by impairing the viability of the sperm and ovum through the alteration of the fallopian tube and uterine fluids. This reduces the chances of the ovum and sperm from meeting and impedes fertilization. The IUD may also prevent implantation, and causes a foreign body reaction with an increase in leucocytes.

Efficacy

The IUD is from 98% to nearly 100% effective in preventing pregnancy, depending on the device. Newer IUDs like the Copper T 380 have a failure rate of less than 1 per 100 after 1 year of use. The Gynefix has a cumulative pregnancy rate of 0.5 at 3 years.

Disadvantages

- ❖ Menorrhagia
- ❖ Dysmenorrhoea
- ❖ Slightly increased risk of ectopic pregnancy if there is an IUD failure
- ❖ Increased risk of pelvic infection (see p. 145)
- ❖ Expulsion of the IUD
- ❖ Perforation of the uterus, bowel and bladder
- ❖ Malposition of the IUD
- ❖ Pregnancy caused by expulsion, perforation, or malposition.

Advantages

- ❖ Effective immediately
- ❖ No drug interactions
- ❖ Reversible and highly effective
- ❖ Not related to sexual intercourse

Absolute contraindications

- ❖ Pregnancy
- ❖ Undiagnosed genital tract bleeding; once the cause has been diagnosed and treated an IUD may be inserted
- ❖ Previous ectopic pregnancy
- ❖ Pelvic or vaginal infection; once treated an IUD may be fitted
- ❖ Abnormalities of the uterus, e.g. bicornuate uterus
- ❖ Allergy to components of IUD, e.g. copper
- ❖ Wilson's disease
- ❖ Heart valve replacement or previous history of bacterial endocarditis because of increased risk of infection
- ❖ HIV and AIDS because of reduced immune system and increased risk of infection

Relative contraindications

- ❖ History of pelvic infection
- ❖ Dysmenorrhoea and/or menorrhagia
- ❖ Fibroids and endometriosis
- ❖ Penicillamine treatment may reduce the effectiveness of copper (Guillebaud, 1993).

Range of method

There are six intrauterine devices available in the UK. Three different IUDs are shown in Fig. 8.1 and Table 8.1 lists all six together with details of their life span and construction.

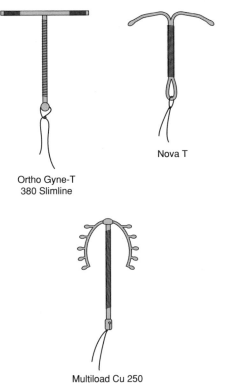

Ortho Gyne-T
380 Slimline

Nova T

Multiload Cu 250

Fig. 8.1   Three different intrauterine devices. (Reproduced from *Women's Sexual Health*, G. Andrews (ed.), 1996, Baillière Tindall.)

Side effects

❖ Menorrhagia
❖ Dysmenorrhoea.

Decision of choice

The decision of which IUD to insert will depend on the woman and the size of her uterus. The Multiload CU250 and Multiload CU375 are suitable for women with a uterine length over 7 cm, while the Multiload CU250 Short is suitable for a woman with a uterine length of 5–7 cm. The Novagard is suitable for a uterine length of over 5.5 cm, while the Nova T and Ortho Gyne T380 Slimline are suitable for a uterine length of over 6.5 cm. The Gynefix is a frameless implant with no arms (Wildemeersch *et al.*, 1994) which is fitted with an anchoring system to

Table 8.1 Names and details of life span and construction of six intrauterine devices.

Device	Life span	Construction
Multiload	3 years	Vertical stem 3.6 cm in length; 250 mm^2 of copper wound around stem
Multiload CU250 Short	3 years	Vertical stem 2.5 cm in length; 250 mm^2 of copper wound around stem
Multiload CU375	5 years	375 mm^2 of copper wound around stem
Novagard	5 years	200 mm^2 of copper wound around stem
Nova T	5 years	200 mm^2 wound around stem
Ortho Gyne T380	8 years	320 mm^2 wound around stem and 30 mm^2 of copper on the distal portion of each arm
Gynefix	5 years	Frameless IUD with 6 copper tubes each 5 mm in length and 2.2 mm in diameter with total 330 mm^2 of copper wound around stem and arms.

fix the antifertility components of the device permanently to the fundus of the uterus. It has been developed to reduce the risk of expulsion, and to lessen symptoms such as pain and bleeding, which are reasons for early removal.

Research (Sivin & Stern, 1994) has shown that IUDs similar to the Ortho Gyne T380 Slimline, which were compared to the levonorgestrel IUD, have low pregnancy rates and low and declining rates of side effects, including pelvic infection. Research undertaken in Africa has confirmed that the pregnancy rates with Copper T380s are low (Farr & Amatya, 1994; Farr et al., 1996). Complications are most likely to occur at the insertion of an IUD. Perforation of the uterus, vasovagal shock, expulsion of the IUD, pelvic infection, pain and bleeding may occur following insertion or in the first year of use. The Ortho Gyne T380 Slimline IUD is licensed for 8 years, which means that the risks associated with insertion are decreased, as it does not require frequent changing. Research (Allison, 1995) has been undertaken on the long-term use of the Nova T beyond its licence of 5 years. When the Nova T was left in situ a further 3 years it showed a low pregnancy and expulsion rate and a low rate of removal because of infection.

If a woman wishes to have an IUD fitted then the most suitable IUD will be one which has a long licence and high efficacy, resulting in lower risk of pelvic infection, expulsion and perforation. However the IUD inserted will also depend on the size and shape of a woman's uterus, and the inserter will take into consideration all these factors when choosing which device to fit.

IUD counselling

When counselling a woman about an intrauterine device you should take a full past and present medical history, which will help to exclude any absolute contraindications. Your discussion of the efficacy and risks of an IUD should include the following points.

1. Clients should be aware that their periods may be heavier and more painful. Menstrual periods may improve within a few months after insertion. If they are already painful and heavy another form of contraception may be more suitable like the Levonorgestrel IUS.

2. The risk of pelvic infection is slightly increased at insertion and for the first 20 days following it. Research has shown (Farley *et al.*, 1992) that the risk of pelvic inflammatory disease (PID) was six times higher during the first 20 days following insertion, which emphasizes the need for screening and follow up, and suggests that limiting changing of IUDs will reduce the risk of infection. This research showed that there was a small or no risk of PID associated with long-term use of IUD, and that exposure to sexually transmitted diseases is the major cause of pelvic inflammatory disease rather than the type of IUD. An IUD will not protect any woman against sexually transmitted diseases and HIV, so these issues need to be approached with her. If your client is not in a permanent relationship and wishes to have an IUD inserted then her risk to exposure to sexually transmitted diseases may be higher and this should be discussed along with safer sex.

   This research indicates the necessity for routine screening. Routine screening for chlamydia should be undertaken at a consultation prior to insertion for all women, so that the results are available at insertion. If a woman is having a post-coital IUD inserted, then prophylactic antibiotics should be given and screening for chlamydia should be performed at insertion. However any woman who is experiencing symptoms of a sexually transmitted disease, e.g. dyspareunia (painful sexual intercourse), offensive discharge or on vaginal examination is found to have cervical excitation, pelvic pain or cervicitis, should have full screening for sexually transmitted diseases performed. If this is unavailable she should be referred to a genito-urinary medicine clinic.

   You should encourage your client to attend earlier following an IUD insertion if she experiences any signs of vaginal infection such as abdominal pain along with pyrexia, so that full infection screening can be performed and antibiotics given early to prevent pelvic infection.

3. You should discuss with your client the risk of expulsion of the IUD. This is most likely to occur following insertion, which is why it is important for your client to attend a follow up consultation in 4–6 weeks after insertion. It is also important to teach her to check her IUD threads every month after her menstrual period. If she can feel the end of the IUD device, which will feel like the end of a match stick, she should be advised to use alternative contraception and return to see you.

4. There is a rare risk that during insertion the IUD may perforate the uterus or cervix. If your client experiences low abdominal pain which

continues following insertion with no improvement she should be advised to see a doctor.

5. Efficacy should be discussed with women, as no form of contraception is 100% effective against pregnancy. If an IUD fails then there is a risk that a pregnancy may be an ectopic pregnancy, so you should advise women to return early so this can be excluded. If she experiences low abdominal pain which is persistent and either missed or scanty periods she should seek help immediately.

An IUD is usually inserted at the end of a menstrual period as the cervix is slightly opened at this time, making insertion easier. An IUD may be inserted up to 5 days after the earliest calculated day of ovulation as post-coital contraception. Following delivery of a baby a woman can have an IUD fitted 6 weeks postnatally. After a miscarriage or a termination of pregnancy then an IUD may be inserted immediately if the pregnancy was less than 12 weeks.

It is a good idea to encourage women to eat prior to an IUD insertion, as they will then be less likely to feel faint following insertion. Many women allow themselves little or no time to recover from insertion. Following insertion they may experience cramp-like period pains and it can be helpful to warn them to allow more time for themselves and perhaps organize for someone else to pick up their children or leave work earlier that day.

The areas to be covered at counselling are summarized in Box 8.1

Insertion procedure

Prior to insertion the chlamydia result should be checked, information about the last menstrual period obtained to exclude an already present pregnancy, and

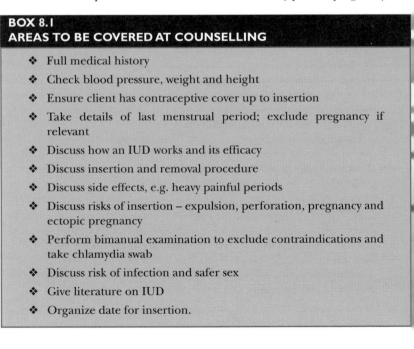

BOX 8.1
AREAS TO BE COVERED AT COUNSELLING

- ❖ Full medical history
- ❖ Check blood pressure, weight and height
- ❖ Ensure client has contraceptive cover up to insertion
- ❖ Take details of last menstrual period; exclude pregnancy if relevant
- ❖ Discuss how an IUD works and its efficacy
- ❖ Discuss insertion and removal procedure
- ❖ Discuss side effects, e.g. heavy painful periods
- ❖ Discuss risks of insertion – expulsion, perforation, pregnancy and ectopic pregnancy
- ❖ Perform bimanual examination to exclude contraindications and take chlamydia swab
- ❖ Discuss risk of infection and safer sex
- ❖ Give literature on IUD
- ❖ Organize date for insertion.

8: The intrauterine device (IUD)

a pregnancy test performed if required. Research (Guillebaud, 1993) has shown that if mefenamic acid 500 mg is given orally prior to insertion there is a reduction in pain following insertion of an IUD. Women should empty their bladder prior to insertion as this will make it easier for the inserter to feel the uterus abdominally and more comfortable for the woman.

During the IUD insertion procedure your client may like to have someone to hold her hand and comfort her – this may be you or a friend or partner. Prior to insertion a bimanual examination will be performed by the inserter to ascertain the size, position and direction of the uterus, and to check that there is no tenderness.

The skill and expertise of the inserter will help reduce any problems and side effects. However if a woman would like to have local anaesthetic to reduce pain or has had problems with an IUD in the past, then this can be given with lignocaine gel or a paracervical block using lignocaine. She may need to be referred to a hospital clinic which specializes in difficult insertions and removals. If lignocaine is given via a paracervical block then the lignocaine ampoule should be warmed to 37°C as this has been found to reduce the pain of the initial injection (Davidson, 1992).

Insertion of an IUD is performed by a 'non-touch technique' so a clean pair of gloves should be used following bimanual examination. A sterile speculum is inserted into the vagina and the cervix is located; this is cleaned with sterile cotton wool and antiseptic solution. A uterine sound is inserted into the uterus via the cervical canal to measure the length, direction and patency of the uterus. This may cause cramp-like period pains which should diminish when the uterine sound is removed. The cervix may be stabilized by Allis forceps or a tenaculum so that the IUD may be inserted more easily; these may cause some discomfort as the cervix is very sensitive. Next the IUD is inserted through the cervical canal into the uterus. The threads of the IUD are shortened once it is in position and are tucked up behind the cervix. If there are any problems with an insertion then your client should be referred to a specialist in IUDs.

Following insertion you should encourage your client to lie down and rest. Analgesia may be required for period pains. Sanitary towels should be used initially to reduce the risk of infection and because tampons may catch on the IUD threads which have not yet softened. Tampons may be used with the next menstrual period. Your client may experience bleeding initially. This is a good time to remind her of any initial problems and when to return, for example if she experiences a change in her normal vaginal discharge or persistent abdominal pain.

You should teach your client how to check her IUD threads and encourage her to perform this after each menstrual period. It is helpful to show your client a picture of the type of IUD she has fitted, and how long it should remain *in situ*. Up-to-date written information should be given along with relevant telephone numbers of where to get help if needed. The IUD is effective immediately so no additional contraception is required. An IUD procedure takes usually 10 minutes.

You will need to see your client in 4–6 weeks for an initial follow up after insertion.

Vasovagal and anaphylaxis attacks

Vasovagal and anaphylaxis attacks are usually rare, however it is important to have emergency equipment and clear guidelines available for such events. Your

8: The intrauterine device (IUD)

client may feel sweaty and complain of feeling faint or sick. She may look pale and her pulse may be slower. If the IUD insertion procedure is still in progress then this should be stopped, and the woman should be laid in supine position with her head lowered and feet raised. If bradycardia persists then slow intravenous atropine 0.3–0.6 mg may be required. If the woman has difficulty breathing and there is loss of consciousness and absence of a carotid pulse, her airway should be maintained by using a Brook airway or Laerdal pocket mask and emergency services phoned and help summoned. She should be laid in the left lateral position, and if there is no central pulse then 1/1000 of adrenaline 0.5–1.0 ml may be given by deep intramuscular injection. If there is no improvement this may be repeated at 10 minute intervals to the maximum of three doses. If required cardiopulmonary resuscitation should be commenced. The woman should never be left unattended at any time.

Subsequent visits

You should see your client 4–6 weeks post IUD insertion to examine and discuss any problems she may have. Details of the last menstrual period should be taken, along with any problems she has experienced. You should ask about any pain or difficulties having sexual intercourse, can her partner feel the IUD threads? Has she been able to check her threads herself? This information will help you when you examine your client, as it will give you signs for infection and you will be able to re-teach your client how to check her threads if she is unable to do so. Your client should be examined with a speculum first so that the IUD threads may be observed. If the IUD threads appear too long they may be shortened. If a cervical smear is required then this may be taken at this time. After the speculum examination a bimanual examination should be performed. If the tip of the IUD can be felt in the cervical os, which might not have been seen on speculum examination, then the IUD is too low in the uterine cavity and will need to be removed and a new device fitted. The cervix should be checked for cervical excitation by moving it gently from side to side. If pain is experienced whilst this is performed this may indicate infection or an ectopic pregnancy. If any signs of vaginal or pelvic infection are observed then you should refer your client to a genitourinary medicine clinic for full infection screening if unavailable on site.

If there are no problems then the IUD should be checked every 6 months, but you should advise your client to return earlier if she experiences any problems.

Research (Bontis *et al.*, 1994) into copper IUDs and their pregnancy rates concluded that the pregnancy rate seemed to reduce if women were taught to self check their IUD's threads and had frequent follow up appointments.

Removal procedure

An IUD may be removed at any time if a client does not mind becoming pregnant. However if she wishes to avoid becoming pregnant alternative contraception should be commenced at least 7 days prior to removal. If an IUD is being changed and a problem arises which prevents insertion of a new device, then emergency hormonal contraception may be indicated for sexual intercourse prior to removal of the old device.

An IUD is removed by inserting a speculum into the vagina and locating the cervix, from which the IUD threads should be visible. Spencer Wells forceps are applied to the IUD threads and gentle traction is applied. The IUD should slowly descend into the vagina. If this does not happen then this may be because the IUD has become embedded in the uterus, and you should refer your client to a specialist doctor experienced in difficult removals.

It is usually advised that IUDs are removed 1 year after the menopause, because there is concern that an IUD may cause pyometra (pus in the uterus) (CSAC, 1993b).

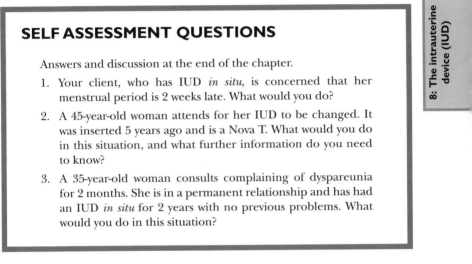

SELF ASSESSMENT QUESTIONS

Answers and discussion at the end of the chapter.

1. Your client, who has IUD *in situ*, is concerned that her menstrual period is 2 weeks late. What would you do?

2. A 45-year-old woman attends for her IUD to be changed. It was inserted 5 years ago and is a Nova T. What would you do in this situation, and what further information do you need to know?

3. A 35-year-old woman consults complaining of dyspareunia for 2 months. She is in a permanent relationship and has had an IUD *in situ* for 2 years with no previous problems. What would you do in this situation?

8: The intrauterine device (IUD)

Problems encountered

❖ *LOST THREADS:*

If you or your client are unable to feel the IUD threads this may indicate that the IUD has been expelled or that the IUD has moved within the uterus, or perforated the uterus taking the threads with it. You should advise your client to use alternative contraception as she may be at risk of pregnancy. However she may already be pregnant and a pregnancy test should be performed to exclude this, along with details of her last menstrual period and any signs of pregnancy which may be experienced. Extrauterine pregnancy should be excluded first by ultrasound scan. If your client has an intrauterine pregnancy and wishes to continue with the pregnancy the IUD may be left in situ if it is too difficult to remove. She should be advised that there is an increased risk of spontaneous abortion, premature labour or stillbirth. The IUD should be located after the birth if there are no complications.

If your client is not pregnant then the threads may be found using either Spencer Wells forceps or a thread retriever like the Retrievette or the Emmett (Bounds et al., 1992b). If the threads are still lost then an ultrasound should be performed to locate the position of the IUD. If the IUD is found to be correctly positioned in the uterus then no further action is required. However if it is not seen then a straight abdominal X-ray should be performed to exclude perforation.

❖ **PERFORATION:**

If an IUD perforates the uterus then it may also perforate the bowel or bladder, and an ultrasound and X-ray will need to be performed to locate the device and laparoscopy performed to remove the device.

Perforation is rare and more common in post partum lactating women who have IUDs fitted. It is important to encourage women to return if they have any pain or discomfort which persists following insertion.

❖ **INFECTION:**

If a woman complains of any change in her normal discharge such as vaginal itching, soreness, offensive and/or increased discharge or pain, then this should be investigated fully. If screening for all genital infections is unavailable then you should refer women to their local genitourinary medicine clinic where screening for chlamydia and sexually transmitted diseases will be performed.

Clients may wish to reduce the risk of infection by using spermicides. Spermicides act as germicides, killing bacteria, and may be used throughout the cycle. Safer sex should be discussed. Women may choose to use an IUD as a method of contraception and a condom to protect them against infection.

❖ **ECTOPIC PREGNANCY:**

If a woman complains of low abdominal pain which may be associated with a light, scanty or missed period then an ectopic pregnancy should be excluded. A pregnancy test and bimanual examination will need to be performed to confirm diagnosis; if this is confirmed then she will need to be referred to her local hospital for emergency treatment. If diagnosis is unconfirmed by examination and pregnancy test then an urgent ultrasound will be performed to further exclude any likelihood of an ectopic pregnancy.

❖ **PREGNANCY:**

If a woman is pregnant with an intrauterine pregnancy and has an IUD in situ, *then if she wishes to continue with the pregnancy the IUD should be removed if the pregnancy is less than 12 weeks' gestation, the threads are visible and removal offers no resistance. There is a risk of spontaneous abortion if the IUD is removed but this is greater if the IUD is left in* situ. *It is not always possible to remove the IUD. Removal should only be attempted by an experienced doctor following discussion with the client.*

❖ **PAIN OR BLEEDING:**

If a woman complains of pain or bleeding with an IUD then this should be investigated fully first to exclude infection, perforation or ectopic pregnancy. Details about the bleeding pattern or pain should be ascertained, and a pregnancy test performed along with a bimanual examination and cervical smear test, screening for infection and ultrasound scan. If the pain continues and infection, perforation and ectopic pregnancy have been excluded then appropriate analgesia may be given, or the IUD may be changed. Changing an existing IUD to a different type of IUD may be a possible solution.

❖ *ACTINOMYCES-LIKE ORGANISMS (ALOs):*

Actinomyces-like organisms are bacteria found in women with IUDs in situ by cytologists when cervical screening is performed. If a woman is asymptomatic e.g. she does not complain of pain, dyspareunia, or an increase in vaginal discharge then the IUD may be removed and sent for culture, with the IUD threads removed and a new IUD fitted. If the culture is negative to actinomyces then a follow up smear should be repeated. However if the culture is positive to actinomyces then she will require antibiotic therapy which should be advised by the microbiology department.

If your client is asymptomatic the presence of actinomyces-like organisms does not necessitate removal of the device, however careful counselling including symptoms which do necessitate removal and follow up should be discussed. After full counselling your client will be able to make an informed decision about whether she wishes to have the IUD removed or left in situ. This decision should be documented in her notes.

The future

With research now indicating that IUDs may be left *in situ* longer, with less risk of infection and expulsion, it is likely we will see licensing for IUDs being lengthened.

Sexuality and anxieties

Women who choose the IUD as their form of contraception do so often because it is 'out of sight and out of mind', meaning it requires little compliance or motivation from the woman and once *in situ* 'can be forgotten'. With an IUD there is no disruption to sexual intercourse, and therefore no loss of spontaneity. However there are still many misconceptions held about IUDs by both men and women. Many people believe that the IUD causes infertility, infection and is an abortifacient. With such strong inaccurate views held it is not surprising that many woman do not consider it as an initial form of contraception; this highlights the need for comprehensive counselling.

Many women are unaware of new IUDs with higher efficacy and longer life spans, which may take some women over difficult periods where other contraception is contraindicated and the menopause is not too far off! Women may be concerned over the pain of insertion of an IUD. The use of pre-insertion analgesia and local anaesthetic can help to reduce this; however the comfort and support of a nurse or a partner is vital.

A large proportion of women who have completed their families and do not wish to have any more choose to have an IUD fitted; this may be because they see the risks of an IUD as relative now that their family is complete.

8: The intrauterine device (IUD)

ANSWERS TO SELF ASSESSMENT QUESTIONS

1. **Your client, who has IUD *in situ*, is concerned that her menstrual period is 2 weeks late. What would you do?**

   It is important to exclude pregnancy when your client has a delayed menstrual period. Details of the last episode of sexual intercourse and last menstrual period should be ascertained, and a pregnancy test performed if required. If your client is at risk of pregnancy and the test is negative then she will need to have a bimanual examination and ultrasound scan to exclude extrauterine or intrauterine pregnancy. If these are all negative then your client may be reassured that she is not pregnant. If the test is positive then she will need to have a bimanual examination and ultrasound scan to exclude extrauterine pregnancy. If the pregnancy is an ectopic pregnancy then your client will need to be referred to the local hospital for emergency surgery. Once an extrauterine pregnancy has been excluded depending on how your client feels about the pregnancy then this will determine her care. If she does wish to proceed with the pregnancy and wishes to have a termination of pregnancy then the IUD may be removed at the time of the termination procedure. If your client wishes to continue with the pregnancy and is under 12 weeks gestation then the IUD may be removed following discussion of the risks with her, if removal requires no resistance.

2. **A 45-year-old woman attends for her IUD to be changed. It was inserted 5 years ago and is a Nova T. What would you do in this situation, and what further information do you need to know?**

   On discussion with the woman it may be decided to leave the IUD *in situ* longer. She should be given as much information about keeping devices in past their licence so that she can make an informed decision.

   It may be useful to find out when the woman's mother went through the menopause as this may give an indication as to when she may do so. This will give a very rough idea on how long she will require contraception for. It is also important to find out how she feels about pregnancy and whether it will cause her more anxiety by not changing the IUD.

3. **A 35-year-old woman consults complaining of dyspareunia for 2 months. She is in a permanent relationship and has had an IUD *in situ* for 2 years with no previous problems. What would you do in this situation?**

   It is important to find out more about the dyspareunia. Has

there been a change in the women's discharge? Does she have pain at any other time? How long has she had dyspareunia? Can she describe the pain when she gets it?

She will need to be examined to exclude infection and to check the IUD. A bimanual and screening for all infections should be performed. If these are unavailable then she will need to be referred. Until infection has been excluded she should be advised to use condoms to protect her partner against infection.

Once infection has been excluded and the IUD has been checked to be in the correct position, then other causes of dyspareunia need to be investigated. There may be a psycho-sexual aspect to the dyspareunia which may need to be explored. Has the woman's relationship changed? Has she had dyspareunia before? Given time this client may be able to talk about this difficult area.

8: The intrauterine device (IUD)

THE INTRAUTERINE SYSTEM (IUS)

Introduction and history

In 1995 a new method of contraception, known as Mirena, was launched onto the UK market. This product was developed by The Population Council and Leiras, a Finnish pharmaceutical company. Mirena is a Levonorgestrel-releasing intrauterine system (IUS). The development of the IUS has been a long process; the initial idea was considered in 1970. The process began with the development and production of a device which had a sleeve which released constant levels of the hormone Levonorgestrel over a long period of time.

Explanation of the method

The intrauterine system (abbreviated to IUS) has a plastic T-shaped frame similar to a Nova T IUD but has a steroid reservoir around the vertical stem of the device containing the hormone Levonorgestrel. The device is 32 mm in length and 4.8 mm in diameter. It is inserted through the cervical canal into the uterus, where it sits releasing 20 µg of Levonorgestrel over 24 hours. Mirena is impregnated with barium sulphate which makes it radio-opaque, and has a shelf life of 3 years. At present Mirena is licensed for 3 years use in the UK but has a recommended duration of use of 5 years (see Fig. 9.1)

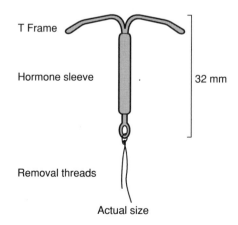

T Frame

Hormone sleeve

32 mm

Removal threads

Actual size

Fig. 9.1 Levonorgestrel IUS. (Reproduced from *Women's Sexual Health*, G. Andrews (ed.), 1996, Baillière Tindall.)

The IUS prevents pregnancy by the suppression of the endometrium, making it unfavourable to implantation. In some women the IUS reduces ovarian function. It also causes the cervical mucus to thicken, making it impenetrable to sperm, and there is a foreign body reaction to the presence of the IUS.

Efficacy

The IUS has a mean failure rate of less than 0.2 per 100 woman years (Luukkainen, 1993). Published comparative multicentre trials, which have covered more than 10 000 woman years (Luukkainen, 1993), have shown that the pregnancy rate has remained very low every year in the studies lasting more than 5 years.

Disadvantages

- ❖ Amenorrhoea
- ❖ Irregular bleeding
- ❖ Body of the IUS device is wider than other IUDs which means that dilatation of cervix may be required
- ❖ Expulsion of the IUS
- ❖ Perforation of the uterus, bowel and bladder
- ❖ Malposition of the IUS
- ❖ Pregnancy caused by expulsion, perforation or malposition
- ❖ Slightly increased risk of ectopic pregnancy if there is an IUS failure
- ❖ Not suitable for post-coital use.

Advantages

- ❖ Reduction in menorrhagia
- ❖ Reduction in dysmenorrhoea
- ❖ Oligomenorrhoea and amenorrhoea
- ❖ High efficacy
- ❖ Reversible
- ❖ Unrelated to sexual intercourse.

Absolute contraindications

- ❖ Pregnancy
- ❖ Undiagnosed genital tract bleeding; once the cause has been diagnosed and treated an IUD may be inserted
- ❖ Heart valve replacement or previous history of bacterial endocarditis because of increased risk of infection
- ❖ Congenital or acquired uterine anomaly which distorts the fundal cavity
- ❖ Suspected or confirmed uterine or cervical malignancy

❖ Recent trophoblastic disease
❖ Serious side effects occurring on the COC which are not due to oestrogen
❖ Present liver disease, liver adenoma or cancer
❖ Present thrombophlebitis or thromboembolic disorder.

Relative contraindications

❖ Chronic systemic disease
❖ Drugs which may interfere with the efficacy of the Mirena, e.g. enzyme-inducing drugs (Leiras, 1995)
❖ Risk factors for arterial disease
❖ Past or present severe arterial disease
❖ Severe lipid abnormalities
❖ Recurrent cholestatic jaundice
❖ Sex steroid-dependent cancer, e.g. breast cancer
❖ Functional ovarian cysts which have required hospitalization
❖ Previous ectopic pregnancy.

Range of method

At present there is only one IUS available – Mirena.

Decision of choice

Women who are interested in having an IUS fitted should be carefully counselled about the side effects of the IUS. Functional ovarian cysts have been noted to be between 10 and 12% with the IUS (Robinson *et al.*, 1989); most were asymptomatic and resolved spontaneously. The most common side effect with Mirena is irregular bleeding patterns, while other side effects were found initially in the first few months following insertion. Research (Andersson *et al.*, 1994; Sivin & Stern, 1994) has shown that the IUS significantly reduces bleeding and spotting, and is particularly useful for women requiring contraception and treatment for menorrhagia and dysmenorrhoea (Bounds *et al.*, 1993).

When the IUS is removed fertility returns to normal immediately and menstruation occurs within 30 days (Hollingworth & Guillebaud, 1994).

Side effects

❖ Some women may develop functional ovarian cysts
❖ Breast tenderness
❖ Acne
❖ Headaches
❖ Bloatedness

9: The intrauterine system (IUS)

❖ Mood changes
❖ Nausea
❖ Irregular bleeding
❖ Amenorrhoea.

Drugs which affect the efficacy of the IUS

The efficacy of the IUS may be affected by liver enzyme-inducing drugs such as Rifampicin, carbamazepine, phenytoin and barbiturates, although this has not been studied (Leiras, 1995).

IUS counselling

As with any method of contraception, the more information given to a client will not only ensure that he or she chooses the best method, but increases their future acceptability of the method. When counselling your clients about the IUS it is important to obtain a full medical history to exclude any contraindications. The side effects and efficacy of the IUS should be discussed, along with your client's contraceptive history. It is important that up until insertion a reliable form of contraception is used as the IUS is not licensed as a post-coital form of contraception.

Many women will choose to have the IUS inserted because of its high efficacy and therapeutic effects on menorrhagia and dysmenorrhoea, even if it may make their already present acne or breast tenderness worse. This is often because they feel that their contraception and periods are the greatest of these problems, and that they will if necessary put up with other problems to alleviate these. However a woman who has very severe pre-menstrual problems and no problems with dysmenorrhoea or menorrhagia may find a new IUD more suitable, such as an Ortho Gynae T380, as this will not increase her pre-menstrual symptoms.

To increase the acceptability and continuation rates with the IUS it is important to discuss the hormonal side effects such as mastalgia, headaches, acne, hirsutism and mood swings. Clients may choose to accept these side effects because of the advantages of the IUS, however they should also be reminded that the amount of Levonorgestrel received through the IUS is only a fraction of the daily dose received through oral contraceptives so the side effects should be smaller with the IUS than with oral methods.

The IUS may cause oligomenorrhoea or amenorrhoea. There is a total reduction in menstrual blood loss because of the reduction in the thickness and vascularity of the endometrium caused by the presence of the IUS. This means that women may experience shorter, lighter, irregular menstrual periods and spotting. Spotting decreases with use and has been found to be less than 4 days at 6 months of use (Leiras, 1995). Woman should be warned that they may experience amenorrhoea which may cause some women anxiety; others however may see this as an advantage.

The risks of IUS insertion procedure should be discussed along with the choice of having local anaesthetic. It is important to talk about the possible need to dilate the cervix to introduce the IUS device, as this may be more painful than having an IUD device inserted, and occasionally the cervix will not dilate enough to allow insertion of the IUS resulting in failure to fit the device. With all IUD and IUS procedures there is a small risk of perforation of the uterus or cervix, however with an experienced inserter this risk will be lessened. There is a risk of partial or complete expulsion of the IUS, which is why it is important for it to have fundal positioning to reduce this possibility. The IUS has a low contraceptive failure rate, but if there is a method failure the pregnancy may be ectopic (Leiras, 1995). However ectopic pregnancies are rare with the IUS, occurring in only 0.02 per 100 woman years (Andersson *et al.*, 1994; Sivin & Stern, 1994) compared with 1.2–1.6 per 100 woman years for women using no contraceptive method (Andersson *et al.*, 1994).

It is important to counsel your client about the possible risks if she becomes pregnant with an intrauterine pregnancy with the IUS *in situ*. Because of the high efficacy of the device there is limited information available about the outcome of a pregnancy with the IUS. Because of the local exposure to Levonorgestrel of an intrauterine pregnancy teratogenicity and virilization cannot be excluded, and termination of the pregnancy should be discussed. If this is discussed at counselling, then women have the opportunity to think about this issue, and if they hold strong views against abortion they may wish to choose another method.

Prior to insertion of the IUS a bimanual examination should be performed to exclude any abnormalities of the uterine cavity such as fibroids, which will necessitate an ultrasound scan to confirm diagnosis prior to insertion. If a fibroid is causing the uterine cavity to be distorted then the IUS will be contraindicated. Screening for chlamydia should be performed at this examination. If there is any suspicion of a genito-urinary infection full screening should be performed; if this is unavailable then your client will need to be referred to a genitourinary clinic.

Areas to be covered at counselling are summarized in Box 9.1.

IUS insertion procedure

Prior to insertion of the IUS the chlamydia result should be checked, information about the last menstrual period should be obtained to exclude an already present pregnancy, and a pregnancy test performed if required, as the IUS is not licensed as a post-coital contraceptive. Fitting of the IUS is similar to that of the IUD. Research (Guillebaud, 1993) has shown that if mefenamic acid 500 mg is given orally prior to insertion there is a reduction in pain following insertion of an IUD. Women should empty their bladder prior to insertion as this will make it easier for the inserter to feel the uterus abdominally and more comfortable for the woman. Emergency equipment should be available at all IUS and IUD insertions (see p. 147)

During the IUS insertion procedure your client may like to have someone to comfort her. Prior to insertion a bimanual examination will be performed by the inserter to ascertain the size, position and direction of the uterus, and to check that there is no tenderness.

Your client may like to have local anaesthetic to reduce pain, as the cervix may need to be dilated to fit the IUS. Anaesthesia can be given with a paracervical block using lignocaine. If lignocaine is given via a paracervical block then the lignocaine ampoule should be warmed to 37°C as this has been found to reduce

---

BOX 9.1
AREAS TO BE COVERED AT COUNSELLING

- ❖ Full medical history
- ❖ Check blood pressure, weight and height
- ❖ Ensure client has contraceptive cover up to insertion
- ❖ Take details of last menstrual period; exclude pregnancy if relevant
- ❖ Discuss how an IUS works and its efficacy
- ❖ Discuss insertion and removal procedure
- ❖ Discuss side effects, e.g. amenorrhoea, irregular menstrual cycle
- ❖ Discuss risks of insertion – expulsion, perforation, pregnancy and ectopic pregnancy
- ❖ Perform bimanual examination to exclude contraindications and take chlamydia swab
- ❖ Discuss safer sex
- ❖ Give literature on IUS
- ❖ Organize date for insertion.

---

the pain of the initial injection (Davidson, 1992). As an IUS insertion may involve dilatation of the cervix to introduce the device, the procedure should be carried out by an inserter who has received further training in IUS insertion and paracervical anaesthesia.

Insertion of an IUS is performed by a 'non-touch technique' so a clean pair of gloves should be used following bimanual examination. A sterile speculum is inserted into the vagina and the cervix is located; this is then cleaned with sterile cotton wool and antiseptic solution. A uterine sound is inserted into the uterus via the cervical canal to measure the length, direction and patency of the uterus. This may cause cramp-like period pains which should diminish when the uterine sound is removed. The cervix may be stabilized by Allis forceps or a tenaculum so that the IUS may be inserted more easily; these may cause some discomfort as the cervix is very sensitive. As the introducer to the IUS is wider than other IUDs – it is 4.8 mm in diameter compared with a Nova T which is 3.7 mm in diameter – Hegar dilators may need to be used to dilate the cervix to Hegar 5 or 6 in diameter. This may be uncomfortable and local anaesthetic can help to alleviate this discomfort. Next the IUS is inserted through the cervical canal into the uterus. The threads of the IUS are shortened once it is in position and are tucked up behind the cervix. Fundal positioning of the IUS is extremely important to reduce the risk of expulsion and to ensure the endometrium has full exposure to the progestogen in the device and maximum efficacy is obtained.

Following insertion you should encourage your client to lie down and rest. Analgesia may be required for period pains. Sanitary towels should be used initially to reduce the risk of infection and because tampons may catch on the IUS threads which have not yet softened. Tampons may be used with the next menstrual period. Your client may experience bleeding initially; this is a good time to remind her of any initial problems and when to return, for example if she experiences a change in her normal vaginal discharge or persistent abdominal pain.

You should teach your client how to check her IUS threads and encourage her to perform this after each menstrual period. It is helpful to show your client a picture of the IUS and give up-to-date written information along with relevant telephone numbers of where to get help if needed. It is recommended that the IUS is fitted within the first 7 days of the onset of menstruation, when no additional contraception is required. An IUS procedure takes usually 10 minutes. The batch number of the IUS device and expiry date should be recorded in the woman's notes. You will need to see your client in 4–6 weeks for an initial follow up after insertion. Your client should be advised to return earlier if she experiences pain, unusual vaginal discharge, or pyrexia.

The IUS can be inserted immediately following a first trimester abortion, and should be inserted 6 weeks post partum following delivery. The IUS is not recommended as a first choice of contraception for women breast feeding.

IUS removal procedure

Removal of the IUS is the same as removing an IUD, and as fertility returns immediately contraception should be discussed prior to removal, e.g. diaphragm should be taught and fitted prior to removal if wanted.

Subsequent visits

Following insertion of the IUS an examination should be performed 4–6 weeks later, when blood pressure and weight should be taken. Details about menstrual cycle and any problems experienced should be ascertained. If your client has had amenorrhoea since fitting then a pregnancy test should be performed to exclude pregnancy, however if there are no symptoms and the device is *in situ* then you can reassure your client. A speculum and bimanual examination should be performed to check that the device is correctly positioned. The IUS threads should be visible on speculum examination. If the end of the IUS device is felt (it feels like the end of a match stick), then the device is partially expelled. This is a good opportunity to show your client how to check her threads for the IUS if she is unable to do so.

If there are no problems and the device is correctly positioned then you should see your client in 6 months' time to check the device. However you should remind your client when to return early, for example if she experiences any persistent abdominal pain, unusual discharge, pyrexia or symptoms of pregnancy, or if she is in any way concerned.

Problems encountered

❖ *LOST THREADS:*
  If you or your client are unable to feel the IUS threads this may indicate that the IUS has been expelled or that it has moved within the uterus or perforated the uterus taking the threads with it. You should advise your client to use alternative contraception as she may be at risk of pregnancy. However she may already

be pregnant and a pregnancy test should be performed to exclude this, along with details of her last menstrual period and any signs of pregnancy which may be experienced. Extrauterine pregnancy should be excluded first by an ultrasound scan. If your client has an intrauterine pregnancy then careful counselling will need to be given.

If your client is not pregnant then the threads may be found using either Spencer Wells forceps or a thread retriever like the Retrievette or the Emmett (Bounds et al., 1992b). If the threads are still lost then an ultrasound should be performed to locate the position of the IUS. If the IUS is found to be correctly positioned in the uterus then no further action is required. However if it is not seen then a straight abdominal X-ray should be performed to exclude perforation.

❖ *PERFORATION:*
If an IUS perforates the uterus then it may also perforate the bowel or bladder, and an ultrasound and X-ray will need to be performed to locate the device and laparoscopy performed to remove the device. It is important to encourage women to return if they have any pain or discomfort which persists following insertion.

❖ *ECTOPIC PREGNANCY:*
If a woman complains of low abdominal pain which may be associated with a light, scanty or missed period then an ectopic pregnancy should be excluded. A pregnancy test and bimanual examination will need to be performed to confirm diagnosis. If this is confirmed then she will need to be referred to her local hospital for emergency treatment. If diagnosis is unconfirmed by examination and pregnancy test then an urgent ultrasound will be performed to further exclude any likelihood of an ectopic pregnancy.

❖ *PREGNANCY:*
If a woman is pregnant with an intrauterine pregnancy and has an IUS in situ *then careful counselling will need to be given about the possible risk of teratogenicity and virilization in the fetus, due to local exposure to Levonorgestrel. Due to lack of clinical experience with pregnancies with an IUS* in situ *information is limited, and a termination of pregnancy should be discussed with your client.*

❖ *PAIN:*
If a woman complains of pain or bleeding with an IUS then this should be investigated fully to exclude infection, perforation, ectopic pregnancy. Details about the bleeding pattern and pain should be ascertained, and a pregnancy test performed along with a bimanual examination and cervical smear test, screening for infection and an ultrasound scan.

❖ *ACTINOMYCES-LIKE ORGANISMS (ALOs):*
Actinomyces-like organisms are a bacteria found in women with IUSs in situ *by cytologists when cervical screening is performed. If a woman is asymptomatic,*

e.g. she does not complain of pain, dyspareunia or an increase in vaginal discharge, then the IUS may be removed and sent for culture, with the IUS threads removed and a new IUS fitted. If the culture is negative to actinomyces then a follow up smear should be repeated. However if the culture is positive to actinomyces then she will require antibiotic therapy which should be advised by the microbiology department.

However if your client is asymptomatic the presence of actinomyces-like organisms does not necessitate removal of the device. However careful counselling including symptoms which do necessitate removal and follow up should be discussed. After full counselling your client will be able to make an informed decision about whether she wishes to have the IUS removed or left in situ. This decision should be documented in her notes.

❖ *HEAVIER OR INCREASED MENSTRUAL BLEEDING:*

Heavier or increased menstrual bleeding may indicate a partial expulsion of the IUS as the endometrium may not be having full exposure to Levonorgestrel; there will also be a decrease in efficacy of the device. You should advise your client to use alternative contraception, e.g. condom. She should have a bimanual and speculum examination and a pregnancy test to exclude partial or complete expulsion and pregnancy. If this is not excluded then an ultrasound should be performed to locate the device.

9: The intrauterine system (IUS)

SELF ASSESSMENT QUESTIONS

Answers and discussion at the end of the chapter.

1. A 24-year-old woman consults requesting contraception after being refused a sterilization because of her age. She has three children and has had two miscarriages. None of her pregnancies have been planned and she finds it difficult to remember to take pills. What forms of contraception would be suitable for her?

2. What are the advantages of the IUS to a woman?

3. Who would be most suitable for IUS, and who do you think would be less suitable for an IUS and why?

The future

The IUS has widened the field of contraception: not only does it offer excellent reversible contraception, but has been shown to have qualities that make it extremely effective in the treatment of menorrhagia. Research is currently being undertaken into the properties of the IUS as a form of hormone replacement therapy (HRT). Initial research has shown that the Levonorgestrel IUS offers an alternative route for giving progestogen for hormone replacement treatment

(Andersson *et al.*, 1992; Raudaskoski *et al.*, 1995; Suhonen *et al.*, 1996). However the Levonorgestrel IUS is not licensed for use as a form of HRT and is not licensed for the treatment of menorrhagia if contraception is not required. If the Levonorgestrel IUS is used for these indications it must be on a 'named patient basis' and the medico-legal responsibility is taken by the prescriber (for further information see Ferner, R.E., 'Prescribing licensed medicines for unlicensed indications,' *Prescriber's Journal* **36**, No. 2).

Sexuality and anxieties

With the introduction of the IUS the field of contraception has widened considerably. Not only does Mirena offer an extremely effective form of contraception but it offers many women treatment for dysmenorrhoea and menorrhagia; for many of these women the only relief of these symptoms would have been to have a hysterectomy. Mirena also offers women a suitable reversible option to sterilization, and has given women who are unable to use combined oral contraception another acceptable choice.

Many women who consult requesting Mirena have complex gynaecological and sexual histories – they perceive the IUS as being the answer to all their problems, which it may well be! Often these women have tried all methods of contraception in an effort to solve their problem, with no success. However some of these problems may be of a psychosexual nature, which the IUS will not alleviate. Given time these anxieties may surface; if however they are not expressed, they may appear as feelings of dissatisfaction with the method.

ANSWERS TO SELF ASSESSMENT QUESTIONS

1. **A 24-year-old woman consults requesting contraception after being refused a sterilization because of her age. She has three children and has had two miscarriages. None of her pregnancies have been planned and she finds it difficult to remember to take pills. What forms of contraception would be suitable for her?**

   From this history the client is looking for a method of contraception which has a high efficacy and which does not require compliance, as she finds it difficult to remember to take oral contraception. There are several methods available to her which fit this description – Depoprovera, IUDs and the IUS. Careful counselling should be given about each method and a detailed medical history taken, so an informed decision may be made by the client. Some women may choose not to have Depoprovera because of the requirement of having injections every 11–12 weeks. An IUD like an Ortho Gynae T380, which has an 8-year licence, may be a good choice or an IUS; both offer high efficacy and little client compliance.

2. **What are the advantages of the IUS to a woman?**
The main advantages of the IUS to a woman are that her periods will become less painful and lighter; she may also experience no periods. If a woman has experienced anaemia from heavy periods this will also be alleviated. The IUS offers highly effective contraception with very low pregnancy rates, with the added benefit of being completely reversible. Lastly, the IUS requires little compliance from a woman and is unrelated to sexual intercourse.

3. **Who would be most suitable for an IUS, and who do you think would be less suitable for an IUS and why?**
Those most suitable for the IUS are women:

❖ Requesting a method of contraception for a 3-year period or more

❖ Who want a method with a high efficacy; they may have had a contraceptive failure or do not wish to become pregnant

❖ Who may suffer from heavy or painful periods

❖ Who may be unable to use other methods of contraception because of contraindications, e.g. they have focal migraines and are unable to have the COC, or they may be unable to have the IUD due to heavy periods.

Women who are less suitable for the IUS include those who have experienced side effects with progestogen methods. These women may find the menstrual disturbances unacceptable. Some women find it disturbing to have amenorrhoea as this usually is an indicator of pregnancy. Women are unable to have the IUS fitted if they are pregnant, have undiagnosed genital tract bleeding, or have a suspected malignancy or liver disorder. Women who have an abnormality of the uterus which distorts the uterus may be unable to have the IUS because the device may be expelled more easily. Women with circulatory disorders, thromboembolic disease, heart valve replacement and history of bacterial endocarditis should not have an IUS because they are absolute contraindications. Other contraindications are women who have had recent trophoblastic disease, chronic systemic disease or who are taking drugs which may interfere with the efficacy of the IUS.

9: The intrauterine system (IUS)

EMERGENCY CONTRACEPTION

❖ **Introduction and history**
❖ **Hormonal contraception**
❖ **Intrauterine contraceptive devices**

INTRODUCTION AND HISTORY

The first emergency contraceptives used to prevent pregnancy were douches; understandably these were not very successful. In the 1960s the first hormonal post-coital preparations used contained oestrogen only. This was replaced in 1983 by Yupze regimen, which contains oestrogen and progestogen and must be taken within 72 hours of unprotected sexual intercourse. An intrauterine device may be inserted as a post-coital method, but this is not generally as well known as the Yupze regimen with the general public or professionals.

Emergency contraception is usually referred to by men and women as the 'morning after pill'. This term has created huge problems because many people have mistakenly believed that they may only obtain emergency contraception the day after unprotected sexual intercourse, when in fact they have a much longer time period!

In 1992 the government produced a white paper called *The Health of the Nation*, which identified certain areas of concern. It set targets, one of which was to reduce conceptions in women under 16 years of age by 50% by the year 2000 (Department of Health, 1992a). The reduction of conceptions can only be achieved by increased education about contraception and sexual intercourse, and when emergency contraception can be taken and where it is available. Following the publication of this document in 1995 the Health Education Authority and The Family Planning Association ran a campaign which included an information pack on emergency contraception in an effort to increase awareness amongst health professionals. However many studies have shown that the message about emergency contraception is still failing to get through to many men and women. Of 177 women seeking an abortion (Gooder, 1996) only 13 women had used emergency contraception and a further four had been unable to obtain it, even though knowledge of emergency contraception was over 80%. However other studies have shown greater deficiencies in knowledge (Crosier, 1996): of 97% of surveyed women who had heard of 'the morning after pill' less than a quarter were able to give the correct time limits for emergency contraception, and only 14% had heard of it through a health professional. Another survey (Hughes & Myers, 1996) concluded that although there was high level of knowledge about the existence of emergency contraception this understanding was incomplete, and only 12% were aware that an IUD could be used as a post-coital method. This indicates how important it is for health professionals to constantly revise and update women on post-coital contraception at every available opportunity.

Emergency contraception has two main methods: hormonal contraception and intrauterine contraception.

HORMONAL CONTRACEPTION

Explanation of the method

The Yuzpe regimen is at present the only licensed form of hormonal post-coital contraception. It prevents pregnancy in a number of ways depending where in the cycle it is administered. It can prevent or delay ovulation if given early in a menstrual cycle, which is why careful condom use must be adhered to for the rest of the cycle as further unprotected sexual intercourse may be at greater risk of pregnancy. It is thought that the Yuzpe regimen causes the genital tract fluid and uterine fluid to become hostile to sperm and ovum, hindering ovum transport. If the Yuzpe regimen is administered after ovulation it causes the endometrium to become unfavourable to implantation, and impairs the corpus luteum function which shortens the luteal phase.

Efficacy

The efficacy of the Yuzpe regimen varies between 95 and 99% in preventing pregnancy (Kubba, 1995), with the lower efficacy rate applying to mid cycle unprotected sexual intercourse which has the greatest risk of pregnancy.

However not all episodes of unprotected sexual intercourse result in pregnancy. It is estimated from an analysis of published trials that this regimen's efficacy reduces the probability of pregnancy by 75% (Trussell et al., 1996). Although this is a great reduction in the risk of pregnancy, it is no replacement for effective ongoing contraception. An episode of unprotected sexual intercourse on any day in the menstrual cycle has an overall risk of pregnancy of 2–4% (Trussell & Stewart, 1992; Kubba, 1995) and will be higher around ovulation at between 20 and 30% (Kubba, 1995).

Disadvantages

❖ Does not provide future contraception
❖ Next menstrual period may be early or delayed
❖ Nausea and vomiting.

Advantages

❖ Effective in preventing pregnancy
❖ Under the woman's control.

Absolute contraindications

❖ Pregnancy
❖ Present focal migraines
❖ Current hepatocellular jaundice
❖ Sickle cell crisis
❖ Current active arterial disease
❖ Active porphyria. ⎫ (Guillebaud, 1997)

Relative contraindications

❖ Past history of arterial disease (Guillebaud, 1997)
❖ Past history of venous thrombosis
❖ Previous ectopic pregnancy
❖ Breast feeding women
❖ More than 72 hours has elapsed since unprotected sexual intercourse.

10: Emergency
contraception

Range of method

The Yuzpe regimen is produced in four tablets made of the hormones oestrogen and progestogen, each tablet containing 0.05 mg of Ethinyloestradiol and 0.25 mg of Levonorgestrel. It is available in the form of Schering PC4 for post-coital use, with an instruction leaflet.

The first dose of the Yuzpe regimen should be commenced within 72 hours of the earliest episode of unprotected sexual intercourse, and the second dose taken 12 hours later. Although this regimen is only licensed for 72 hours it may be given later (Guillebaud, 1995). Although there is no research into the efficacy of the Yuzpe regimen administered after 72 hours, the efficacy will be lower and the responsibility for this unlicensed use will be the prescriber's. This should be discussed fully with the client, along with the alternative choice (an IUD) so that she is able to make an informed decision.

Other hormonal methods

At present the only hormonal method licensed for post-coital use is the Yuzpe regimen. Other methods have been used which have the advantage of not containing oestrogen, but these methods involve complicated regimens and high doses of hormones and are unlicensed for post-coital use.

Levonorgestrel method

This involves taking 0.75 mg of Levonorgestrel within 48 hours of the earliest episode of unprotected sexual intercourse and a further 0.75 mg of Levonorgestrel 12 hours later. Each dose can only be given by taking 25 tablets Microval or Norgeston. The only research undertaken was a randomized study comparing the Levonorgestrel method and the Yuzpe regimen. This study gave an efficacy of 97.6% (Ho & Kwan, 1993) for the Levonorgestrel method compared with 97.4% for the Yuzpe regimen, and concluded that the Levonorgestrel method had a lower incidence of side effects like nausea, vomiting and fatigue.

Other unlicensed progestogen regimens have been used but the research involved has had small numbers of subjects, resulting in limited clinical experience.

Side effects

- ❖ Nausea
- ❖ Vomiting
- ❖ Fatigue
- ❖ Headaches
- ❖ Dizziness
- ❖ Breast tenderness.

Decision of choice

The hormonal method of post-coital contraception is a safe effective method. The decision of which method to choose is made once a careful history has been taken and detailed counselling given. It is important to ascertain when unprotected sexual intercourse has taken place; if this is beyond 72 hours then the Yuzpe regimen will be contraindicated. If a woman has an absolute contraindication to the hormonal method then an IUD should be considered. Women wishing to use the IUD as a method of contraception may have this fitted as an emergency method, however it is important to remember that occasionally an IUD is unable to be fitted and if this is the case it may be more likely to occur with nulliparous women. Another factor to remember when choosing which method to use is the risk of genitourinary infection which may be the result of the unprotected sexual intercourse. Because of this factor if the episode is within 72 hours then taking the hormonal method may be of less risk to the woman than fitting an IUD (see Fig. 10.1).

How to take the Yuzpe regimen

The hormonal post-coital method is prescribed as Schering PC4. Schering PC4 contains four tablets. Two tablets should be taken within 72 hours from the earliest episode of unprotected sexual intercourse, and the remaining two tablets taken 12 hours later. As the Yuzpe regimen can make women feel nauseated, it is a good idea to advise them to take the tablets with or after food, or with an antiemetic like Motilium (Domperidone).

If the client vomits within 2 hours after taking the first dose of Schering PC4 then she should take the second dose of pills immediately if within the 72 hours and be advised to return and obtain a further two pills to complete the course. If a client vomits within 2 hours of the second dose she should be advised to return for a further two pills. If a woman suffers from severe vomiting then an IUD may need to be considered.

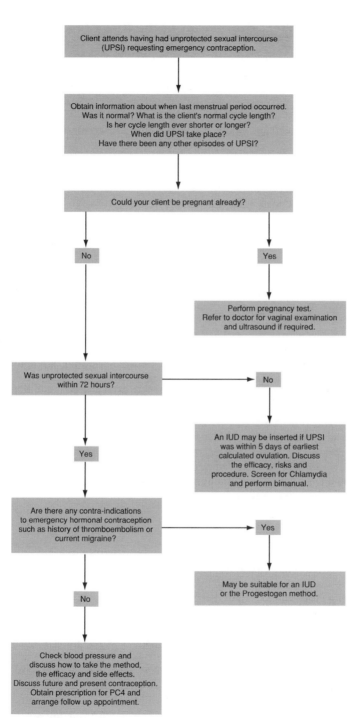

Fig. 10.1 Emergency contraception – management plan.

Drugs which affect the efficacy of the Yuzpe regimen

Drugs which reduce the efficacy of the Yuzpe regimen are enzyme-inducing drugs like Rifampicin. In this situation the woman should be advised to increase the number of tablets she takes so that she takes three tablets initially and a further three 12 hours later, so that she has taken a total of six tablets of Schering PC4 (Belfield, 1997). It is now believed that there is no need to increase the dosage of the Yuzpe regimen if a woman is taking antibiotics (Belfield, 1997).

Counselling

Women who attend for emergency contraception are often very anxious and embarrassed; they may show varying emotions from anger to guilt. Sexual intercourse may not have been with consent, and she may feel shocked and distressed. Often the situation women find themselves in feels threatening to them, and their feelings of anger and guilt, etc. are aimed at you. You may come across women who have difficulty in answering some of the personal questions you need to ask. 'Why do you need to know that?' is not an uncommon response. It is important to allow enough time for this consultation and explain why you need to ask such personal questions. It is also a good idea to allow your client time to read through up-to-date literature about emergency contraception beforehand so that you can build on this knowledge and answer any questions this may initiate.

Often clients fail to tell you about earlier episodes of unprotected sexual intercourse as they do not feel they are at risk of pregnancy from these episodes. Women often believe that unprotected sexual intercourse around the end of their menstrual period will be safe, so this can be a good opportunity to explain about ovulation and how it is possible for sperm to live in the body for up to 7 days (Guillebaud, 1993). If your client has had earlier unprotected sexual intercourse then the hormonal method will be contraindicated but it may be possible to fit an IUD if it is within 5 days of calculated date of ovulation. It is useful when taking details about episodes of earlier unprotected sexual intercourse to chart these on a menstrual calendar along with details of when the first day of the last menstrual period occurred and length of normal menstrual cycle; this will also make calculating ovulation easier. Often whilst you are doing this it triggers clients' memories and they remember further episodes of unprotected sexual intercourse.

If there is any doubt that your client's last menstrual period was not normal then a pregnancy test should be performed to exclude pregnancy. Some women mistakenly believe that emergency contraception will be effective in preventing an existing pregnancy.

When counselling men and women about emergency contraception it is important to discuss the efficacy and side effects of post-coital contraception. Sometimes women decide not to have emergency contraception after they have received counselling; this usually happens when the woman is in a stable relationship and willing to accept the risk of pregnancy, or if the risk is low. Occasionally it is not possible to give post-coital contraception because the woman has had multiple episodes of unprotected sexual intercourse which exceed 72 hours and are beyond 5 days of calculated ovulation so an IUD is unable to be inserted. This situation is often made worse if the woman has had unprotected sexual intercourse with someone other than her regular partner. As health professionals you want to make 'everything better'. This is a situation when you are unable to do this, and this can not only be very difficult for the client but also for the nurse. What you may find hardest is that you can give no guarantees – you cannot reassure the woman that she won't become pregnant, because there is a real risk that she may become pregnant. You also need to approach the issue of safer sex and contraception, which may at this time be an area she has not thought of. Listening to the woman's distress and anxieties are the main functions of the nurse. It is often hard not to falsely reassure a woman in this situation, but being there and listening to the pain your client is suffering are far more important to her. An appointment should be made after your client's estimated next menstrual period so that a pregnancy test can be performed; if possible this appointment should be with you.

Sometimes the request for emergency contraception has been precipitated by rape. Shock may stop a woman from attending early for emergency contraception, which may mean that an IUD is indicated or that you are unable to give emergency contraception. It is vital that a woman has screening for all genito-urinary infections and HIV from a specialist clinic. Rape counselling should be offered. Women may feel that they do not want this at the time, but information and telephone numbers should be given in case they wish to follow this up in the future.

Many different women and men attend for emergency contraception. They may be women in their forties whose unprotected sexual intercourse may cause a change in their contraceptive practice to a permanent method like sterilization in the future; they may feel that they should know better and be embarrassed. Other clients may be young men and women who may be under the age of 16 and recently commenced sexual activity. They may be anxious that the information they give may not stay confidential, embarrassed and humiliated by the personal questions that are asked. Many younger clients feel that they will be judged by the health professionals they see. It has usually taken a great deal of courage for them to attend, and the impression they gain from this encounter will establish whether they attend in the future. Their confidentiality should be respected unless the health, safety or welfare of someone other than the client is at serious risk (BMA *et al.*, 1993). Occasionally young clients are being sexually abused and if given time for a rapport to establish they may return to confide in you.

A full medical history of the client and family should be completed to exclude any contraindications such as present focal migraines. If a client has previously had emergency contraception it is useful to know if she had any problems such as vomiting, etc. so that appropriate advice can be given. If a woman has used emergency contraception repeatedly because of a contraceptive failure or because no contraception has been used, then future contraception should be discussed carefully. If your client has had a contraceptive failure teaching them how to avoid this in the future will help reduce the necessity of emergency contraception in the future.

It is extremely important that women continue to use either a condom or abstain until their next period as hormonal emergency contraception will not stop a woman from becoming pregnant in the remaining part of the cycle. If a woman has a further episode of unprotected sexual intercourse then she may be more at risk of pregnancy, because the Yuzpe regimen can delay ovulation, resulting in this episode now being when she is ovulating! Women should be advised that if this situation occurs they need to return for further treatment. There is often a great deal of anxiety about giving repeated doses of hormonal emergency contraception but as along as the latest episode is within 72 hours and there is no other contraindications then the Yuzpe regimen may be prescribed.

ACTIVITY

Do you know where your clients can receive emergency contraception if you are unavailable? What about weekends and bank holidays?

Blood pressure, height and weight should be checked, a pelvic examination is not required with the hormonal method unless pregnancy is suspected or screening for infection is suspected. Anyone who has unprotected sexual intercourse puts themselves at risk of sexually transmitted disease and HIV, and if full infection screening is unavailable then they should be referred to their local genitourinary medicine clinic.

When giving emergency contraception to clients exploration of their attitudes to pregnancy and discussion of the possible failure of emergency contraception is important. At present there is no evidence to show that hormones used as post-coital methods carry any risk of teratogenicity (Kubba, 1995), however no one can guarantee a normal outcome to any pregnancy. Information is being gathered about the outcome of pregnancies following failed hormonal postcoital contraception (Cardy, 1995), and recorded by the Clinical and Scientific Committee of the Faculty of Family Planning and Reproductive Healthcare.

You should advise your client that her next menstrual period may be early, on time or later than expected. If it is not a normal period or is absent she should return with a urine sample so that a pregnancy test can be performed. There is a risk in early pregnancy of an ectopic pregnancy. If a woman experiences abdominal pain she should be advised to seek medical attention. It is good practice to offer women the opportunity to return 3–4 weeks later; this gives you the opportunity to review any problems with contraception.

As clients are often very anxious when they consult all the information you give should be backed up by up-to-date information, as they are more likely because of their anxiety to forget details. It is useful to have up-to-date information available of other local clinics who offer emergency contraception. If for example you give emergency contraception on a Friday and the client vomits and requires a second dose of pills, it is useful to give them addresses of alternative clinics if you are not available on the Saturday. It is a good idea to advertise this information in your waiting room and make it available to other staff in case they receive telephone enquires.

The areas to be covered at counselling are summarized in Box 10.1.

Follow up appointment

You should offer to see your client 3–4 weeks following post-coital contraception to check that she has had a normal menstrual period. If this is shorter or lighter

---

BOX 10.1
AREAS TO BE COVERED AT COUNSELLING

- ❖ First day of last menstrual period and details of menstrual cycle length
- ❖ Was her last menstrual period normal – is there any possibility that she may already be pregnant? Do you need to perform a pregnancy test?
- ❖ Time and date of earliest unprotected sexual intercourse
- ❖ Has your client any contraindications to emergency contraception?
- ❖ What contraception was used? Is your client happy to continue with this method or does she want another method?
- ❖ Has she had emergency contraception before? Did she have any problems with it, e.g. vomiting?
- ❖ Record blood pressure
- ❖ Does your client understand how to take the emergency contraception and know when she needs to return?
- ❖ Has your client read and been given up-to-date information about emergency contraception, and does she have contact numbers if she vomits or has a problem?

---

than normal a pregnancy test should be performed to exclude pregnancy. It is important to ask if any side effects have been experienced, e.g. vomiting, which may affect the efficacy of this method. Alternative contraception should be discussed at counselling so that it can, if it is a hormonal method, be commenced day 2 of the next period. This is to determine that this menstrual period is normal. The COC should be commenced on day 2 of a normal menstrual period with additional precautions required for 7 days. The POP should be commenced on day 2 of a normal menstrual period, with additional precautions required for 7 days (Guillebaud, 1995).

INTRAUTERINE CONTRACEPTIVE DEVICES

Explanation of the method

An IUD works as a post-coital method by preventing implantation and may also block fertilization. As pregnancy and implantation does not occur until 5–7 days after fertilization, this means that the IUD does not act as an abortifacient.

Efficacy

The IUD is almost 100% effective in preventing pregnancy post-coitally.

Disadvantages

- ❖ Slightly increased risk of ectopic pregnancy if there is an IUD failure
- ❖ Increased risk of pelvic infection
- ❖ Expulsion of the IUD
- ❖ Perforation of the uterus, bowel and bladder
- ❖ Malposition of the IUD
- ❖ Pregnancy caused by expulsion, perforation or malposition
- ❖ Minor surgical procedure.

Advantages

- ❖ Effective in preventing pregnancy
- ❖ Unrelated to partner
- ❖ IUD may be kept *in situ* and used as a form of contraception for the future
- ❖ Longer time span of up to 5 days.

Absolute contraindications

- ❖ Pregnancy
- ❖ Present pelvic, vaginal infection although an IUD may be inserted in special circumstances with antibiotic cover
- ❖ Undiagnosed genital tract bleeding.

Relative contraindications

- ❖ Past history of ectopic pregnancy, although the IUD may be inserted and removed following the next menstrual period
- ❖ Past history of pelvic infection
- ❖ Heart valve replacement or previous history of bacterial endocarditis; because of increased risk of infection an IUD may be inserted with antibiotic cover.

Range of method

The type of IUD usually used post-coitally is a Nova T, but a Multiload or Ortho Gyne T380 Slimline may be used.

Side effects

- ❖ Menorrhagia
- ❖ Dysmenorrhoea
- ❖ An IUD may be difficult to fit in nulliparous women.

Decision of choice

An IUD may be fitted as a form of emergency contraception up to 5 days after the calculated date of ovulation. It provides contraception for the rest of the month, and if a woman wishes can either be left *in situ* after her next menstrual period or be removed. Women who have a contraindication to the hormonal method may be able to have an IUD fitted, along with women who cannot accept the failure rate of the hormonal method.

Counselling

Women who have a post-coital IUD fitted may be more anxious than women having routine IUDs fitted, which can make insertion difficult. As they have had less time to prepare themselves for the procedure, it is important to allow them time to ask any questions and discuss the insertion procedure, risks, efficacy and advantages and disadvantages of the IUD. You should complete a full medical history which will enable you to eliminate any contraindications to the procedure, and with the aid of a menstrual calendar and information on the first day of the last menstrual period estimate the calculated date of ovulation. If there is any possibility of your client being pregnant you should complete a pregnancy test, and a bimanual examination will need to be performed to exclude pregnancy.

If your client has not eaten recently it is preferable that she has something to eat prior to insertion; this will reduce the chances of her feeling faint. Analgesia may be given, and will be absorbed faster if a client has eaten. Although all this may seem time-consuming it will have the effect of reducing anxiety in the woman which will aid insertion of the device and will reduce pain felt following insertion.

Prior to fitting an IUD screening for chlamydia should be performed. As the result will not be available for the insertion of a post-coital IUD prophylactic antibiotics are recommended. If there are signs of cervical or pelvic infection full screening for infection is recommended, especially in the case of rape, which may necessitate referral to a genitourinary medicine clinic (GUM). When referring your client to a GUM clinic, you may find it possible for the post-coital IUD to be inserted following screening at the clinic.

The IUD procedure is the same as for a routine IUD procedure. Clients should be shown how to check their IUD threads, and be advised that she may experience some bleeding and period-like pains after fitting. She should be encouraged to avoid tampons and use sanitary towels immediately after insertion in case these catch on the threads. If she experiences persistent pain she should be advised to seek medical attention to exclude an ectopic pregnancy. It is vital to give up-to-date literature and emergency telephone numbers to your client. A follow up appointment should be made 3–4 weeks following insertion.

Follow up appointment

You should see your client 3–4 weeks following insertion to check that she has had a normal menstrual period. If this is shorter or lighter than normal a pregnancy test should be performed to exclude pregnancy. If she is having her IUD removed with her period then alternative contraception should be commenced 7 days prior to removal. Hormonal contraception is usually commenced on day

10: Emergency contraception

2 of a period to determine that this is normal. The COC should be commenced on day 2 of a normal menstrual period with additional precautions required for 7 days. The POP should be commenced on day 2 of a normal menstrual period, with additional precautions required for 7 days (Guillebaud, 1995). Once alternative contraception has been established then the IUD may be removed. If however she would like to continue with the IUD as her method of contraception the IUD should be checked, and if there are no problems an appointment should be made for 6 months.

Problems encountered with emergency contraception

❖ *VOMITING WITH THE YUZPE REGIMEN:*
   It is a good idea to try and prevent vomiting prior to it happening. Women should be encouraged to avoid taking the Yuzpe regimen on an empty stomach. An anti-emetic like motilium (domperidone) may be prescribed if vomiting occurs with a repeat dose of the Yuzpe regimen. If vomiting is severe an IUD may need to be considered.

❖ *PREVIOUS USE OF THE YUZPE METHOD IN THE CYCLE AND A FURTHER EPISODE OF UNPROTECTED SEXUAL INTERCOURSE:*
   As long as the second episode of unprotected sexual intercourse (UPSI) is within 72 hours then a second dose of the Yuzpe regimen may be given. It is important to check that the previous dose was taken correctly and no other UPSI has taken place other than the recent episode. If this is the case then an IUD may be indicated if it is within 5 days of the earliest calculated date of ovulation.

❖ *YOUR CLIENT HAS A FOCAL MIGRAINE AND HAS HAD UNPROTECTED SEXUAL INTERCOURSE:*
   A focal migraine is a contraindication to the Yuzpe method, in this instance an IUD may be indicated. The levonorgestrel method may also be prescribed if the episode of UPSI is within 48 hours; this would be given on a named patient basis and would be the prescriber's responsibility. Careful counselling of the client is important for this unlicensed use. However this may be the only choice available to the woman if, for example, there is difficulty fitting an IUD.

SELF ASSESSMENT QUESTIONS

Answers and discussion at the end of the chapter.

1. A woman with a regular cycle of 4/25 days attends requesting emergency contraception. It is 100 hours since the first episode of UPSI, and she is now on day 18 of her cycle. Can you give her emergency contraception?

2. What are the indications for emergency contraception?

The future

There has been a large amount of publicity surrounding emergency hormonal contraception, and whether it should be made available to women through the pharmacist. There are strong opinions (Owen Drife, 1993; Cayley, 1995) for and against deregulating the Yuzpe method. Many people believe that if this method was widely available it would reduce the incidence of unwanted pregnancies and pregnancy terminations. However another view is that by making the Yuzpe method freely available to women, there will a great loss of opportunity to counsel and educate women about contraception and safer sex. A step towards making the Yuzpe method more widely available to women whilst still offering counselling would be to give appropriately trained family planning nurses the authority to prescribe. The debate continues.

Sexuality and anxieties

Men and women consulting for emergency contraception are often extremely anxious. This is exacerbated by meeting someone, often in these circumstances for the first time, to discuss intimate details of their sex life, which can make it a harrowing situation. However, if handled appropriately it can be the beginning of a relationship that gives clients a richer knowledge and awareness of sexual health. In giving an empathetic approach to your clients which does not judge their sexual practices you will encourage them to consult in the future.

An episode of unprotected sexual intercourse (UPSI) often precipitates a change in contraceptive method, although clients often fail to mention this. When changing methods it is useful to ask about UPSI as this may affect when a new method may be commenced and may also mean that emergency contraception can be discussed.

Many women perceive the hormonal method to have more risks than regularly taking the combined pill (Ziebland *et al.*, 1996), and often accept the greater risks of an abortion by avoiding taking it. Young men and women are more likely to take the sort of risks that would require emergency contraception than older clients (Pearson *et al.*, 1995), but are less likely to request it. This may be for a number of reasons, from lack of knowledge of its availability and awareness of its use to concern over confidentiality and fear of a hostile reception. This indicates the need to inform clients about emergency contraception – they may never need the information themselves but may inform a friend! Men should not be forgotten when educating clients about emergency contraception; increasingly they are taking an interest and responsibility for contraception which should be encouraged. Often receptionists are forgotten in our zeal to educate, yet it is important that they are aware of the need of these clients to obtain immediate appointments. It is also important that they are aware of other clinics where emergency contraception is available especially outside normal working hours, as they are most likely to receive telephone requests for this information. Giving emergency contraception can not only save a great deal of anguish over an unwanted pregnancy and abortion, but is also much more cost-effective and has less risk to the health of the woman.

10: Emergency contraception

ANSWERS TO SELF ASSESSMENT QUESTIONS

1. **A woman with a regular cycle of 4/25 days attends requesting emergency contraception. It is 100 hours since the first episode of UPSI, and she is now on day 20 of her cycle. Can you give her emergency contraception?**

   Unfortunately as she is more than 5 days from the earliest calculation of ovulation an IUD cannot be fitted; she would ovulate between days 9 and 13. Because she is now 100 hours since her earliest episode of unprotected sexual intercourse the Yuzpe regimen is contraindicated. You should advise her to return in 2 weeks with an early morning urine specimen if she has not had a normal menstrual period within that time. She should continue to use either condoms or abstain for contraception as it is possible that she may not be pregnant.

2. **What are the indications for emergency contraception?**

   The indications for emergency contraception are:

   ❖ Unprotected sexual intercourse, e.g. condom break or misuse, diaphragm fitted incorrectly, no contraception used, missed pills

   ❖ Rape and sexual assault

   ❖ Recent use of drugs with a teratogenic effect where UPSI has taken place, e.g. cytotoxic drugs, live vaccines such as yellow fever.

FEMALE STERILIZATION

Introduction and history

Female sterilization is the only permanent method of female contraception. It was first mentioned by Hippocrates, but it was not until 1834 that Von Blundell fully described this method. At this time it was an extremely dangerous procedure involving abdominal surgery and hospitalization for long periods. In 1944 Drs Decker and Cherry reported on the successful outcomes of their culdoscopy procedure, which involved reaching the fallopian tubes through the vagina rather than through the abdomen. It was not until 1961 that laparoscopic sterilization was first described by Uchida.

Today female sterilization is performed abdominally by either a mini laparotomy or by laparoscopic sterilization or through the vagina by culdoscopy. It can be performed as a day-care procedure either under a general or local anaesthetic.

Explanation of the method

Female sterilization involves excising or blocking the fallopian tubes which carry the ovum from the ovary to the uterus. This prevents the ovum from being fertilized by sperm in the fallopian tube.

Efficacy

Female sterilization is a highly effective form of contraception with a failure rate of 1–5 per 1000 cases, which translates to an efficacy of 99.4–99.8% per 100 woman years. The effectiveness varies depending which method is used: diathermy and Filshie clips are considered the most effective.

Disadvantages

❖ Involves a surgical procedure and anaesthetic
❖ Not easily reversed.

Advantages

❖ High efficacy
❖ Permanent
❖ Effective immediately.

Contraindications

- ❖ Relationship problems
- ❖ Indecision over the operation by either partner
- ❖ Psychiatric illness
- ❖ Ill health or disability which may increase the risk of the operation.

Relative contraindications

- ❖ Request for sterilization at young age, e.g. under 25
- ❖ Obesity may be contraindication for a laparoscopic procedure.

Range of method

Female sterilization involves excising or blocking the fallopian tubes by:

1. Applying a Hulka or Filshie clip – this flattens and occludes the fallopian tube
2. Drawing up a section of the fallopian tube and applying a Falope ring to the tube
3. Cauterization and diathermy
4. Excising and ligating the fallopian tube.

Some of these methods are shown in Fig. 11.1

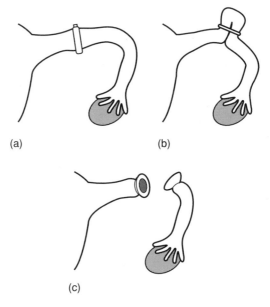

(a)   (b)

(c)

Fig. 11.1 Female sterilization techniques. (a) Filshie clip; (b) Falope ring; (c) tying the ends after the tubes have been cut. (Reproduced from _Women's Sexual Health_, G. Andrews (ed.), 1996, Baillière Tindall.)

11: Female sterilization

Side effects

❖ If there is a method failure then there is a higher risk of ectopic pregnancy

❖ Feelings of grief and loss.

Counselling a couple for female sterilization

Counselling a couple is extremely important for this procedure as it should be considered a permanent method. Careful counselling will also reduce post-operative regret and grief over the loss of fertility which some women experience.

During counselling with the couple you should discuss how they would feel if something happened to their children. How would they feel if something happened to their present partner – would they want children with a new partner? Are they both certain they do not want any more children? There are no set answers to these questions, but they are areas that need to be considered which can be difficult to discuss. It is important to give an unbiased view when discussing sterilization. You may hold personal views yourself about this method but these should not influence the couple in their decision. It is useful to meet the couple together, rather than the woman on her own, as the decision affects both parties and you may get different views and opinions about the decision. However you may wish to complete the medical history with the woman on her own, as there may be details of her personal medical history that her partner is unaware of, e.g. previous abortion.

You should complete a full medical history of your client with special attention to gynaecological history. If for example she suffers from menorrhagia or dysmenorrhoea then this will continue following sterilization. In this situation it may be more appropriate for her to have the levonorgestrel intrauterine system or have a hysterectomy which would treat these symptoms. In the past women often complained that a sterilization caused menorrhagia and dysmenorrhoea; this was more likely due to the fact once they stopped the combined pill, which had reduced these symptoms, they returned to their true cycle following sterilization. Research (Rulin et al., 1993) undertaken to investigate the long-term effect of female sterilization on menses and pelvis pain showed no long-term difference between sterilized and non-sterilized women.

Women should be advised to continue with their present method of contraception until after procedure, so that there is no chance of them being pregnant that cycle. If a woman uses an IUD as her method she should be advised to use condoms for the menstrual cycle prior to the procedure, to ensure that no sperm are present in the fallopian tubes, which could fertilize an ovum that is released shortly after surgery resulting in an ectopic pregnancy.

You should discuss with your clients the efficacy and side effects of sterilization. Sterilization is a very effective form of contraception, but if it fails there is a higher risk of an ectopic pregnancy. You should discuss the difficulties of reversing this procedure so that a couple understand fully the decision they are making. Sterilization should not be performed at a termination of pregnancy or following childbirth as the failure rate is higher due to increased vascularity of

11: Female sterilization

the tissues involved, and there may also be regret of the decision made at this emotional time.

Procedure

Female sterilization is usually performed under general or local anaesthetic and the most common procedure is laparoscopic sterilization. This is where a small incision is made at the umbilicus and the abdomen is filled with carbon dioxide gas. The operating table is tilted backwards, which ensures that all the other organs move away from the uterus. Using the laparoscope the fallopian tubes are located, and either ligated or clips applied. This procedure may be performed as a day case and, depending on home circumstances, it may be possible for the woman to go home that day.

If a woman has had previous gynaecological surgery or is obese it may not be possible to perform a laparoscopic sterilization. In this situation a mini laparotomy may be indicated. This procedure involves a larger abdominal incision and usually requires hospitalization of 4–5 days. After the sterilization most surgeons perform a dilatation and curettage (D&C) to ensure that there is no risk of pregnancy following sexual intercourse prior to the procedure.

Post female sterilization

Following the procedure women may complain of cramp-like period pain for a few days and shoulder pain. This occurs as a result of using carbon dioxide gas and the application of the clips.

Women should be advised to seek medical attention immediately if they experience any signs of pregnancy or miss a menstrual period. This should be investigated to exclude an intrauterine or extrauterine pregnancy.

Women who experience regret over their decision and signs of grief and loss should be offered post-operative counselling, although counselling prior to the operation should reduce this problem.

Reversal of female sterilization

Female sterilization should be considered irreversible. Successful reversal will depend on the type of procedure used when the woman was initially sterilized, her age and the skill of the surgeon performing the reversal. The success in achieving pregnancy following reversal can be between 50 and 90%, depending on the original method used. Following reversal a woman is at a higher risk of ectopic pregnancy, with 3–5% of pregnancies being ectopic (Belfield, 1997).

The methods of sterilization which are most easily reversed are the use of Hulka or Filshie clips, as these flatten the fallopian tubes which can be re-inflated. Cautery and diathermy are the hardest to reverse, and are used less often these days because of the dangers of damaging other organs. The Falope ring can cause a portion of the fallopian tube to necrose, making reversal more difficult.

SELF ASSESSMENT QUESTIONS

Answers and discussion at the end of the chapter.

1. Which women do you think are most suitable for a female sterilization?

2. In what way is age relevant to a request for female sterilization?

Sexuality and anxieties

Women who have a sterilization often feel liberated – they no longer have the anxiety of pregnancy. Often a pregnancy scare precipitates a request for sterilization. This new found freedom from anxiety enables many women to explore their own sexuality, and allow them to enjoy sexual intercourse in a way they have been unable to do before.

ANSWERS TO SELF ASSESSMENT QUESTIONS

1. **Which women do you think are most suitable for a female sterilization?**
   Women who are most suitable for sterilization have completed their families and are in stable relationships. They have considered their future and thought carefully about all the options available to them.

2. **In what way is age relevant to a request for female sterilization?**
   If a woman is under the age of 30 then a request for sterilization needs to be treated with caution. There will be concern that a woman may change her mind and want to have more children, especially if something happens to her present relationship.
   Women who are older in their forties may have only a few fertile years left. It may be more appropriate for these women to choose a method with a high efficacy like Depoprovera, the IUS or an IUD like the Ortho Gynae T380 Slimline. Often women have not considered these methods.

PRECONCEPTUAL CARE

- ❖ **Introduction**
- ❖ **Preconceptual care for men**
- ❖ **Preconceptual care for women**
- ❖ **Genetic counselling**
- ❖ **Socioeconomic influences**
- ❖ **Sexuality and anxieties**

12

INTRODUCTION

Family planning involves preconceptual counselling – many women do not think about becoming pregnant before it's too late! It is important to discuss this subject with women prior to conceiving to reduce the incidence of problems in pregnancy.

PRECONCEPTUAL CARE FOR MEN

Men wishing to conceive should follow certain guidelines:

Alcohol

Alcohol can damage a man's sperm making it harder to conceive. Men are recommended to keep consumption low during this period.

Drugs

Illegal drugs can cause problems in conceiving. This is a good time to try and stop through counselling and support.

Smoking

Smoking can affect a man's sperm. This is a good time to stop smoking as there is an increased risk of cot death if a parent smokes.

PRECONCEPTUAL CARE FOR WOMEN

Women planning to become pregnant should be advised to follow certain guidelines.

Diet

Women should be encouraged to eat a healthy diet low in fat and high in fibre. If they are overweight they should try to reduce their weight well ahead of conceiving, preferably at least 3 months beforehand, so that they do not have depleted stores of vitamins and minerals. Women who are underweight may have difficulty conceiving; they should be advised to eat three meals a day, with snacks in between.

Certain foods should be avoided in pregnancy. These include liver, because of its high level of vitamin A, and foods made with uncooked eggs like mayonnaise and undercooked meat because of the risk of salmonella. Cheeses made with unpasteurized milk and mould ripened cheeses should be avoided, e.g. Brie, Camembert, as they may carry the bacteria *Listeria* which can lead to miscarriage and stillbirth, and serious illness in the unborn baby. Other foods which should be avoided include pâté and cooked chilled chicken, as these also carry the risk of these infections.

Alcohol

Alcohol should be reduced to no more than eight units a week, and no more than two units a day in pregnancy.

Supplements

The Department of Health recommend that women take 400 µg of folic acid prior to conceiving and until they are 12 weeks pregnant to prevent neural tube defects (Department of Health, 1992b).

Toxoplasmosis

This is a parasitic infection which can seriously affect the unborn fetus causing brain damage and blindness. It is a flu-like illness which is contracted through raw meat, cat faeces, sheep and goat milk. Women should be advised to avoid handling cat litter trays, wash their hands when handling animals and wear gloves when gardening.

Smoking

Smoking should be avoided in pregnancy. It is a good idea to try and give up prior to pregnancy. Women who smoke in pregnancy are more likely to have a low birth weight baby which is associated with increased mortality and morbidity in the perinatal period and later in infancy (House of Commons Health Committee, 1990–91).

Rubella

It is vital that women are routinely screened for rubella immunity prior to conceiving. If women are susceptible to rubella they should be immunized and avoid pregnancy for 1 month (Department of Health, 1992c). If a woman is susceptible to rubella and contracts the disease during the first 8–10 weeks of pregnancy this can result in congenital rubella syndrome resulting in damage of 90% of infants. Fetal abnormalities include learning disabilities, cataract, deafness, cardiac abnormalities, intrauterine growth retardation and inflammatory lesion of the brain, lung, liver and bone marrow.

Sickle cell disease and thalassaemia

Women and men who are potential carriers of sickle cell disease and thalassaemia should be routinely screened. Those at risk of sickle cell disease are people of African, West Indian and occasionally of Asian origin, whilst those at risk of thalassaemia are of Mediterranean origin, particularly from Greece, Turkey and Cyprus, and also people from Pakistan and India. Screening and genetic counselling can reduce the incidence of these diseases.

Screening

Women should be encouraged to sort out any health problems they may have before becoming pregnant. Women should make sure that they have had a recent cervical smear and have had regular dental check ups. If there is any likelihood of a sexually transmitted disease being present then full screening should be performed and treatment given.

Drugs and medications

Illegal drugs are harmful to the fetus. Women taking illegal drugs should try to obtain help and counselling prior to conceiving. Legally prescribed drugs should be taken with caution. Doctors and dentists should be advised by women that they are planning to get pregnant. If medications are taken that can be bought over the counter, women should check with the pharmacist that these are safe to take at this time.

GENETIC COUNSELLING

Genetic counselling is offered to couples with a personal or family history of an inherited medical condition, e.g. cystic fibrosis, Down's syndrome. This gives couples the opportunity to make an informed decision following discussion of the facts of the condition concerned and risks involved. Genetic counselling involves discussion of the genetic abnormality and appropriate screening. A full history of the couple involved is taken and a family tree developed which will include the medical history of all family members. From this information the couple will be given an estimation of the risk to future pregnancies of the disorder occurring, and continued counselling and support will be offered so that they are enabled to come to a decision over future pregnancies.

SOCIOECONOMIC INFLUENCES

Many women become pregnant without seeking advice over health beforehand, whilst only a small minority of women actively seek help and advice in planning a pregnancy. As a result it is necessary for health care professionals to approach the subject of pregnancy with women at an appropriate opportunity. This will not only enable women to make adjustments in their diet and have preconceptual screening, but also gives them the time to consider the implications of a pregnancy to their life. This is particularly important for women who are unable to speak English as their first language as they may have less access to literature in their own language. It is often unknown if a women is illiterate, which emphasizes the need to discuss issues verbally and how unreliable it is to expect men and women to read literature provided in waiting rooms.

Often the implications of a pregnancy are not considered until it is too late. In today's financial climate many couples have debts either to credit cards or in the form of negative equity with their mortgage, or perhaps they are unable to sell a property and are living in a property that is now too small for their family. Many men and women no longer feel that their employment is secure; they may not have a permanent contract with their employer or may have a short-term contract, which may cause them anxiety. It may be that by becoming pregnant money will be severely restricted, or employment will be at risk; not all employers are sympathetic to pregnancy. Although there is never a perfect time to become pregnant, a couple may be able to make some provisions for a pregnancy if they give time to consider the implications it will make to them now, or they may decide to accept financial hardship or other problems after discussion with each other. By discussing these issues beforehand and negotiating their future, a couple are less likely to have problems within their relationship after the baby is born.

A pregnancy can cement a relationship, making it closer and stronger, but it can also be the final straw to an unsatisfactory one. Sometimes women mistakenly believe that a pregnancy will solve present relationship problems; usually this is the reverse. Occasionally there are situations when women have been so desperate to have children, because they see their time running out, that they have failed to look at their long-standing relationship with ignored psychosexual problems, which now have to be approached to achieve a pregnancy.

Today many women are the 'breadwinners' in families or their salary is a major part of the family income. This has put restrictions onto the number of children couples choose to have. Women now delay pregnancy till they are older and their career is secure, but this causes many dilemmas as to when the best time for a pregnancy will be. There is of course no 'best time' for a pregnancy and this needs to be explored with clients. It may be that the couple have already left it too late and now have infertility problems, which can cause anger and distress within the relationship at the situation.

Women who are already single parents may be in this situation because of a pregnancy at a young age, a broken relationship, or new phenomenon where women have actively chosen to become pregnant as a single parent. Being a single parent is extremely hard not only for the mother but also for the child involved. Today men and women live further away from their families so there is no close-knit family network to help with upbringing of the child, so it all falls on one person – the mother!

When counselling men and women about preconceptual issues your personal views and attitudes should be hidden, so that a couple are able to come to their own decision. This can be very difficult as couples will often ask whether you have children or what you would do in the given situation. It is important that their decision is their own, as however hard this may be they will be able to accept this more easily in the future if it is their own decision.

SEXUALITY AND ANXIETIES

Today many women delay pregnancy until they are in their thirties or forties and often fail to think about the implications of this decision. Because contraception is so effective, it has helped to delay the decision of pregnancy, creating a dilemma as women now have to actively stop contraception to become pregnant. Women may find it harder to become pregnant as they become older and this can increase their feelings of regret and guilt. Sometimes women find that they have left pregnancy too late and this can cause a great deal of anguish and heartache. With careful counselling these feelings may be able to be explored.

Research shows that women are unaware of the need to take supplementary folic acid (Balen *et al.*, 1994), which emphasizes the need to teach and inform women about preconceptual care. Studies are now being undertaken into maternal nutrition and the aetiology of coronary heart disease. This may help to reduce its incidence in the future (Cresswell, 1996).

12: Preconceptual care

PREGNANCY – WANTED AND UNWANTED

- ❖ **Introduction**
- ❖ **Negative pregnancy test**
- ❖ **Positive pregnancy test**
- ❖ **Symptoms of pregnancy**
- ❖ **Signs of pregnancy**
- ❖ **Pregnancy counselling**
- ❖ **Contraception following abortion**
- ❖ **Methods of abortion**
- ❖ **Sexuality and anxieties**

13

INTRODUCTION

Pregnancy is an area of great concern for women who attend for contraception and family planning advice. Women may consult concerned that they are unable to become pregnant; this may be connected to guilt over previous genitourinary infections or terminations of pregnancy or anxiety over using a method of contraception for a prolonged period like the combined oral contraceptive. Other women may consult unaware that they are at risk of pregnancy and this topic may need to be approached. Some women may already be aware that they are pregnant and require confirmation; they may also have made a decision about the future of this pregnancy. Other women may need time to consider their decision and discuss this with their partner.

If there is any suspicion that a woman may be pregnant a pregnancy test should be performed to confirm this. Sometimes a woman can be so adamant that she is not pregnant that when a pregnancy test disproves this, you can find it hard to believe the test results. A pregnancy test should be performed 1 week after a missed period. It is useful to take a history which should include menstrual cycle length, episodes of unprotected sexual intercourse and contraception, along with any symptoms of pregnancy. Often a woman will tell you openly how she feels about a pregnancy, but if she does not discuss her feelings it is helpful to approach this subject prior to performing the test, as this will help you when you have to give her the results.

ACTIVITY

What abortion facilities are available locally to you? Why not see if you can visit so that you can ensure you are giving up-to-date information.

NEGATIVE PREGNANCY TEST

If a pregnancy test is negative this may be because the test has been performed too early, or because the specimen is too dilute or too old, giving a false negative result. A false negative result can also be due to an ectopic pregnancy or a miscarriage, which will require further investigation if suspected. Details of menstrual cycle, contraception and any episodes of unprotected sexual intercourse should be ascertained. Any complaints of abdominal pain will necessitate further examination. Once an ectopic pregnancy or miscarriage has been excluded a pregnancy test should be repeated in a week's time.

POSITIVE PREGNANCY TEST

If a pregnancy test is positive and a woman wishes to continue with the pregnancy she should self-refer to her general practitioner. However sometimes women are unprepared for a positive result and may need time to discuss this with their partner. An appointment should be made at a convenient time, preferably with you, in the near future. It is useful to work out the gestation of the pregnancy as this will give you an idea of when to see your client for a follow up appointment. You should discuss the options available to her so that she can think and discuss this with her partner. Some women already have a suspicion that they are pregnant and have thought about their options already, basing a decision on their feelings.

It is important to allow a woman time to express her feelings. Many women will ask what you would do in this situation. It is important not to influence a client over her decision and to give non-judgemental counselling. A decision over an unwanted pregnancy is probably one of the hardest dilemmas a woman has to face, yet it will in the long-term be easier if she has been allowed to make this decision herself; an empathetic approach will help her to do this.

SYMPTOMS OF PREGNANCY

Women may complain of the following symptoms of pregnancy:

- ❖ Nausea and vomiting
- ❖ Increased micturition
- ❖ Amenorrhoea
- ❖ Breast changes
- ❖ Skin changes.

SIGNS OF PREGNANCY

Certain signs help to confirm pregnancy.

❖ Positive pregnancy test

❖ Enlarged uterus

❖ Fetal heart sounds can be heard at 10 weeks by sonicaid ultrasonic equipment

❖ Fetal movements felt

❖ Fetal parts felt

❖ Ultrasound can be used to diagnose pregnancy at 6 weeks

❖ X-ray can show fetal skeletons at 14–16 weeks but should be avoided as irradiation can damage the developing fetus.

PREGNANCY COUNSELLING

If a woman feels that she does not want to continue with her pregnancy she has two main options: she can have the baby adopted or have a termination of pregnancy. These days it is rare for women to choose to have their baby adopted and most women will opt for an abortion. In 1991 a total of 179 522 abortions were performed in England and Wales, which was a decrease of 7390 (4%) compared with 1990 (OPCS, 1991).

Women can choose to have an abortion privately or through the National Health Service (NHS). If they wish to have an abortion via the NHS they may need to attend their local family planning clinic or GP for a referral to be made locally. If they choose to have a private abortion this should be a clinic approved by the Department of Health for this procedure.

It is useful to give women a brief outline about the choices of abortion available. It is safer for a woman and less traumatic to have an abortion before 12 weeks. If a woman chooses to have a private abortion then an early abortion before 12 weeks will cost less and can be performed as a day case. Women often mistakenly believe that they will have the abortion at the initial consultation. They should be warned that this appointment usually involves the completing of a medical history. Usually a pregnancy test is repeated and a vaginal examination will be performed to estimate gestation and exclude ectopic pregnancy. Some clinics will perform an ultrasound scan to confirm the gestation of the pregnancy. Women will receive pre-abortion counselling at this appointment and a date for the abortion procedure will be organized. If at any stage a woman wishes to change her mind about her decision she can at any point. As this is such a difficult decision sometimes this does happen, and it is important that she is aware that she has this opportunity.

ACTIVITY

Do you know where women can be referred locally for private and NHS abortions? Do you know how much a private abortion would cost in your area?

An abortion can be carried out under the 1967 Abortion Act if two registered medical doctors find that it is necessary on one or more counts prior to 24 weeks gestation. These are that if the pregnancy were to continue it would involve risk to the life of the woman, or would cause injury to her physical or mental health, or would cause injury to existing children's physical or mental health. Lastly there is a substantial risk of the child being born with physical or mental abnormalities. An amendment to this Act in 1991 reduced the upper limit from 28 to 24 weeks gestation, but in special circumstances this limit does not apply. These circumstances are when the life of the woman is at risk or there is a possibility of permanent injury, or when there is serious fetal handicap.

You should encourage your client to return following the procedure for a follow up appointment so that she can discuss how she feels and any problems can be approached. If the clinic you are referring your client to does not perform opportunistic chlamydia screening then this should be performed along with the provision of contraception. Women may not have considered contraception following the procedure, so it is useful to discuss this and if possible provide it so that it can be commenced immediately after the abortion; this will help reduce any anxiety afterwards. Women often say 'never again' so they are only too happy to discuss contraception, and may choose a different method as they may have a loss of confidence if they have had a method failure.

CONTRACEPTION FOLLOWING ABORTION

The diaphragm and cervical cap should be refitted following an abortion in case a new size is required, whilst the IUS and IUD can be inserted immediately following a first trimester abortion. Following a termination of pregnancy Norplant may be inserted immediately; if inserted later then additional contraception will be required for 7 days. Depoprovera can be given within the first 7 days with no extra precautions required, whilst POP and COC should be commenced the same day or next day with no additional precautions required following a first trimester abortion.

METHODS OF ABORTION

The main methods of abortion are:

1. Surgical abortion which can be carried out by:
   - ❖ Vacuum aspiration
   - ❖ Dilatation and curettage (D&C)
   - ❖ Dilatation and evacuation (D&E)
2. Medical abortion.

Surgical abortion
Vacuum aspiration

This is where the cervix is dilated under general anaesthetic and the contents of the uterus emptied by suction. This is the most widely used method and is carried out before 12 weeks gestation, usually as a day case.

Dilatation and curettage (D&C)

The cervix is dilated and a curette is introduced into the uterus and the contents removed. This is usually carried out under general anaesthetic.

Dilatation and evacuation (D&E)

Again, this is performed under general anaesthetic. The cervix is dilated and the contents of the uterus emptied. Vacuum aspiration is performed after this. This method is usually performed in second trimester abortions and can be undertaken up to 20 weeks, although it is preferable to do this before 16 weeks to reduce the risks of a late abortion.

Medical abortion

A medical abortion can be carried out if a pregnancy is less than or equal to 63 days' gestation, which is confirmed by ultrasound scan. It involves, following counselling, the administration of oral 3 Mifegyne 200 mg tablets on day 1 with an observation period of 2 hours. If the woman vomits within this period then she will have to be referred for a surgical abortion. Some women experience vaginal bleeding and period-like abdominal cramps. Abdominal pain should not be treated with non-steroidal anti-inflammatory drugs (NSAIDS), e.g. aspirin, ibuprofen, mefenamic acid, but other analgesics may be given. Contact telephone numbers are given. If heavy bleeding is experienced or severe pain then clients may need to be admitted earlier.

The client will need to return on day 3, 36–48 hours later, for the insertion of a vaginal prostaglandin called Gemeprost 1.0 mg. She is observed for 6 hours in order to observe blood pressure and any problems which may be experienced. Vaginal bleeding usually begins within 2 hours after administration and may continue for 12 days, gradually lessening. Women will experience abdominal pain, and the abortion should occur within the 6 hour period.

A follow up appointment is carried out 5–9 days after the prostaglandin administration to assess that the treatment has been successful. An ultrasound may be performed if bleeding is still present to exclude pregnancy.

Contraindications

❖ Pregnancy exceeding 64 days' gestation
❖ Suspected ectopic pregnancy
❖ Allergy to mifepristone
❖ Chronic adrenal failure
❖ Long-term corticosteriod therapy
❖ Haemorrhagic disorders
❖ Anti-coagulant treatment
❖ Smokers aged over 35.

13: Pregnancy – wanted and unwanted

Relative contraindications

❖ Asthmatics and chronic obstructive airways disease
❖ Cardiovascular disease
❖ Renal or hepatic disease
❖ Women with prosthetic heart valves
❖ Pregnancies of 56–63 days' gestation.

Side effects

Drug-related side effects:

❖ Nausea
❖ Vomiting
❖ Diarrhoea
❖ Faintness
❖ Hot flushes.

Side effects related to treatment:

❖ Infection
❖ Abdominal pain
❖ Bleeding.

SEXUALITY AND ANXIETIES

An unwanted pregnancy brings many anxieties to women. Even if the decision to have an abortion seems to be right for them, there are inevitably regrets. Women may experience the various stages of grief over their decision – denial, anger, depression and acceptance. How they cope with this loss will depend on the counselling and support they receive. Many women subconsciously remember the date of the abortion and the estimated date of delivery. Often they expect to be chastised for their mistake by professionals, and caution should be taken over women who wish to have a medical abortion or surgical abortion with local anaesthetic who feel that in some way they should suffer for their present situation.

Women who have recurrent abortions may be desperately trying to seek help. There may be relationship problems and/or feelings of loss of self-worth under-lying their cry for attention. Given time and counselling these feelings may be able to be approached and explored.

Sometimes women use unplanned pregnancy and abortion to test their relationship, which can cause problems within it. However it can also bring a couple closer together. Women may become pregnant shortly after this episode, but this time continue with it.

Following an abortion women may choose to change their method of contraception as they may feel a loss of faith in it. A review (Hudson & Hawkins, 1995) of contraceptive practices before and after an abortion showed that following an abortion women changed their method to one with a higher efficacy, generally a hormonal method. Many women following an abortion have a great deal of anxiety over becoming pregnant again, and may consult more with pregnancy scares. Often clients hold misconceptions about abortion; they may believe that their future fertility is affected and this can cause a great deal of guilt.

There has been research (Goldbeck-Wood, 1994) which has shown an association between abortion and breast cancer. However almost all the studies have been retrospective and conflict exists between research teams over causal links (Birth Control Trust, 1994). At the moment the effect of abortion on the risk of breast cancer has not been determined, and further research needs to be undertaken in this area.

THE FUTURE

- ❖ **Introduction**
- ❖ **Current contraceptive research**
- ❖ **Future research**
- ❖ **Problems encountered with contraception**
- ❖ **The future in family planning**

14

INTRODUCTION

Since the mid 1980s there have been many new and exciting developments in the field of contraception. These have included the introduction of Norplant, Mirena and Topaz, the Femidon and the Persona, each bringing a new dimension to an already present method. Norplant and Mirena utilized the properties of the progestogen methods offering new long-term methods to women, whilst Topaz offers a solution to problems with burst condoms that other condoms have not addressed and the Femidon offers women protection against sexually transmitted diseases and HIV. The Persona has made natural family planning and fertility awareness more accessible to women.

All these new developments in contraception illustrate the need to offer a new idea or an improvement on a present method which will be acceptable to its users. Ideally these methods should not only be acceptable, but they should also be 100% effective, reversible with no side effects and inexpensive. Obviously this is the ideal, but in the development of new methods these are still the ultimate aim.

CURRENT CONTRACEPTIVE RESEARCH

Currently research is being undertaken into the development of new plastic male condoms (Short, 1994). It is hoped that these will not only be stronger and less likely to break, but will also be a suitable defence against sexually transmitted diseases and HIV. A new cervical cap has been launched in America called Lea's Shield which can be left *in situ* for 48 hours; research into its efficacy is required. Investigations are underway into the suitability of chlorhexidine as a vaginal spermicide (Chantler, 1992) as this has been shown to be active against HIV.

Research is also underway into the suitability of the intrauterine system as a way of delivering progestogen as part of hormone replacement treatment

(Andersson *et al.*, 1992; Raudaskoski *et al.*, 1995; Suhonen *et al.*, 1996). Clinical trials are underway into a single contraceptive implant, and research is ongoing into the development of monthly injectables which contain oestrogen and progestogen.

Research is being undertaken on a weekly male hormonal injectable which contains testosterone enanthate 200 mg (Bonn, 1996), and trials are being commenced on a male hormonal contraceptive injectable which contains testosterone bucyclate.

All these methods will have taken 5–15 years to develop before they become available to men and women on the market. Some may never make it to the market place and the cost in time and money will be lost.

FUTURE RESEARCH

Research into new contraceptive methods is estimated to cost $20–70 million and development can take 5–15 years (FPA, 1995). Such research may be initiated by the World Health Organization, government-funded bodies, family planning centres, industry, universities or individuals. An example of an individual initiating the development of a method is the new male condom Topaz, which was the idea of Keith Jones (Stuttaford, 1996).

For a method to become licensed in the UK it will have to get over many hurdles. Not only will it require funding, and research volunteers to carry out research on the product, but it will need to adhere to guidelines for licensing the product. Hormonal methods (which includes spermicides but not condoms, diaphragms and IUDs) of contraception are controlled by the Medicines Act which is implemented by the Medicines Control Agency (MCA). An example of the influence of the MCA is with the injectable Depoprovera, which received a short-term licence in the UK following its development in 1962, but was only given a long-term licence in 1984 following pressure from women's groups.

A product is also required to satisfy certain guidelines, for example condoms receive 'CE' marking which means that they meet certain safety regulations from the Central European Directive. Although it is important that products are tested and meet standards, it can also prove costly to the manufacturer. All barrier methods will be required to meet these standards in 1998 if they wish to be sold in the European Community. The contraceptive sponge is no longer manufactured because of changes in production requirements, reducing the choice to women.

All research should follow the guidelines of Good Clinical Practice. Good Clinical Practice (GCP) is a term used in clinical research which was devised to prevent the occurrence of fraud, errors and mistakes by establishing a set of guidelines to adhere to; it also helps to protect the rights of research subjects (Allen, 1991). Clients or patients who take part in research are known as subjects. GCP ensures that subjects who take part in research give informed consent, their participation is voluntary and they have the right to withdraw at any time. Ethics committees ensure that the consent the subject gives is truly informed, and their committee has the rights of the subject as their main objective. No committee member can have any connection with the trial.

GCP entails careful documentation of all research which is audited by the sponsoring company and also by independent personnel. Records of consent, drug accountability and adherence to the research protocol will be carefully checked. GCP helps to prevent fraud in research, for example it ensures that the research includes the number of subjects it purports to have had, that the findings were based on the actual results and that any side effects or complications are documented. Without this careful monitoring of subjects and findings, research can be fraudulent by falsifying subjects and information.

PROBLEMS ENCOUNTERED WITH CONTRACEPTION

Once a method has been licensed in the UK it can still encounter obstacles such as litigation and adverse publicity. Litigation can cost manufacturers considerable amounts of money in defence of lawsuits, and the adverse media attention can affect consumers' confidence in the method and seriously affect sales of the product. Following the 'pill scare' in 1995 over the risk of venous thromboembolism with the combined pill there have been cases where women have claimed against either the doctor or the manufacturer because of the information and care provided. At the same time many women changed their brand of combined pill or even changed their method because of the adverse publicity related to the combined pill. All these circumstances reduce the manufacturer's income, which in turn may reduce funding for future research.

Other problems associated with a method of contraception may not be with the actual product, but with the professional who administers it. An example of this is the problems encountered with Norplant. The distributors strongly recommended that specialized training was undertaken prior to inserting the capsules. However there are now cases of litigation pending over incorrect insertion, and women's view of the method has been clouded by negative publicity.

When undertaking research on a product a specific number of subjects need to be found. This can be not only time-consuming but also difficult. Recruiting subjects for research requires a commitment in their time and the acceptance of an unproven efficacy on a method. A subject needs also to fit the research's criteria, which can be very strict!

It is amazing that with all these problems new methods ever become launched, and it is sad that when they do receive a licence some methods are beset with problems with the media which they do not deserve.

THE FUTURE IN FAMILY PLANNING

Although there are many obstacles to the development of future contraceptive methods, there are many ways in which the role and influence of family planning can expand. Firstly the development of organized education plans in schools on sexual behaviour, pregnancy and contraception, will not only help to reduce pregnancies in the under-16 age group, but may give young people an understanding of the complexities of relationships and greater respect for themselves. Secondly the long-awaited issue of nurse prescribing would, if settled, give appropriately trained family planning nurses wider remit to work at times more acceptable to the public. This would make contraception more accessible to younger clients and working women. Lastly with the changes that have occurred within the NHS it has become increasingly difficult for men and women to receive certain contraception methods outside their own area because of funding restrictions. In an ideal world men and women should be able to consult where they wish for contraception and funding should be given separately.

APPENDIX 1: USEFUL ADDRESSES AND RESOURCES

❖ **Contraception**

❖ **Male condoms**

❖ **Natural family planning**

❖ **Pregnancy/unwanted**

❖ **Nursing organizations**

CONTRACEPTION

1. The Family Planning Association,
    2–12 Pentonville Road,
    LONDON
    NI 9FP

    Telephone 0171 837 5432.
    Telephone 0171 837 4044 Contraception Education Service helpline
    9am–7pm.

2. The Family Planning Association in Northern Ireland,
    113 University Street,
    BELFAST
    BT7 1HP

    Telephone 01232 325488.

3. The Family Planning Association in Scotland,
    Unit 10,
    Firhill Business Centre,
    76 Firhill Road,
    GLASGOW
    G20 7BA

    Telephone 0141 576 5088.

4. The Family Planning Association in Wales,
    4 Museum Place,
    CARDIFF
    CF1 3BG

    Telephone 01222 342766.

5.   Margaret Pyke Centre,
     73 Charlotte Street,
     LONDON
     WIP 1LB

     Telephone 0171 530 3600 for switchboard.
     Telephone 0171 530 3636 for advice sister between 9 am and 4 pm weekdays.
     Telephone 0171 530 3650 for appointments.

MALE CONDOMS

1.   Durex web site addresses for Internet users:
     Consumer site address http://www.durex.com
     Research and development department site address http://www.durex.com/scientific
     Corporate information site address http://www.lig.com

NATURAL FAMILY PLANNING

1.   National Association of Natural Family Planning
     Teachers (NANFPT),
     Natural Fertility Centre,
     Hospital of St John and Elizabeth,
     Brompton House,
     LONDON
     NW8 9NH

2.   Fertility Awareness and Natural Family Planning Service of Marriage Care,
     Clitherow House,
     1 Blythe Mews,
     Blythe Road,
     LONDON
     W14 0NW

     Telephone: 0171 371 1341.

3.   Persona
     Persona information line telephone 0990 134430.
     Persona web site address http://www.unipath.com/persona2

PREGNANCY/UNWANTED

1. British Pregnancy Advisory Service,
   Austy Manor,
   Wootton Warren,
   SOLIHULL,
   West Midlands
   B95 6BX

   Telephone 01564 793225.
   Telephone 0345 304030 for information.

2. Birth Control Trust,
   16 Mortimer Street,
   LONDON
   W1N 7RD

   Telephone 0171 580 9360.

3. Marie Stopes House,
   108 Whitfield Street,
   LONDON
   W1P 6BE

   Telephone 0171 388 0662.
   Telephone 0800 716390 for information.

4. British Pregnancy Advisory Service,
   11–13 Charlotte Street,
   LONDON
   W1P 1HD

   Telephone 0171 637 8962.

5. Pregnancy Advisory Service,
   15 Rosslyn Road,
   East Twickenham,
   MIDDLESEX
   TW1 2AR

   Telephone 0181 891 6833.

NURSING ORGANIZATIONS

1. National Association of Nurses For Contraception and
   Sexual Health (NANCSH),
   c/o EMY Secretarial Services,
   19 Whiteacre Road,
   SOLIHULL
   West Midlands
   B93 9HW

   Telephone 01564 770032

2.   RCN Family Planning Forum,
     Royal College of Nursing,
     20 Cavendish Square,
     LONDON.
     W1M 9AE

     Telephone 0171 409 3333

3.   Scottish Society of Family Planning Nurses (SSFPN),
     9 William Place,
     Scone
     PERTH
     PH2 6TE

4.   NI Association of Family Planning Nurses,
     86 Raven Hill Park Road,
     BELFAST
     BT6 0DG

5.   Association of Psychosexual Nursing,
     c/o Margaret Pyke Research Unit,
     73 Charlotte Street,
     LONDON
     W1P 1LB

APPENDIX 2: FURTHER READING SUGGESTIONS

❖ **For professionals**
❖ **For clients**

FOR PROFESSIONALS

Andrews, G. (Editor) (1997) *Women's Sexual Health.* London: Baillière Tindall.

Belfield, T. (1997) *FPA Contraceptive Handbook,* 2nd edition. London: Family Planning Association (FPA).

Benner, P. (1984) *From Novice to Expert* pp 13–38. California: Addison-Wesley.

Clubb, E. & Knight, J. (1996) *Fertility, Fertility Awareness and Natural Family Planning.* Newton Abbot: David & Charles.

Flynn, A. & Brooks, M. (1988) *Natural Family Planning.* London: Unwin Hyman.

Guillebaud, J. (1993) *Contraception: Your Questions Answered,* 2nd edition. Edinburgh: Churchill Livingstone.

Guillebaud, J. (1997) *Contraception Today,* 3rd edition. London: Martin Dunitz Limited.

Jenkins, D. (1986) *Listening to Gynaecological Patients' Problems.* London: Springer-Verlag.

Kubba, A. (1995) *Emergency Contraception Guidelines for Doctors.* Faculty of Family Planning and Reproductive Health Care of the RCOG.

Loudon, N. (1991) *Handbook of Family Planning,* 3rd edition. Edinburgh: Churchill Livingstone.

Montford, H. & Skrine, R. (eds) (1993) *Contraceptive Care: Meeting Individual Needs.* London: Chapman & Hall.

Schon, D.A. (1987) *Educating the reflective practitioner.* California: Jossey-Bass Inc.

Skrine, R.L. (1989) *Introduction to Psychosexual Medicine for doctors, nurses, students and other health care professionals.* London: Chapman & Hall.

Szarewski, A. (1995) Advice for doctors and nurses when counselling women with regard to Depoprovera. Upjohn Limited.

Tunnadine, P. (1992) *Insights into Troubled Sexuality. A Case Profile Anthology*, revised edition. London: Chapman & Hall.

Van Ooijen, E. & Charnock, A. (1994) *Sexuality and Patient Care: a guide for nurses and teachers*. London: Chapman and Hall.

FOR CLIENTS

Condoms

1.   Durex web site addresses for Internet users:
     Consumer site address http://www.durex.com

2.   Condomania UK Ltd.
     Rivermead,
     Pipers Way,
     THATCHAM,
     Berkshire
     RG19 4EP

     Sales hotline telephone 01635-874393.
     Fax 01635-877622.

3.   Health Education Authority (1996) *Gay Men and Safer Sex*. London: Health Education Council.

Natural family planning

Care line on Persona for women:

Telephone 0345-447744.

Contraception

Szarewski, A. & Guillebaud, J. (1994) *Contraception: A User's Handbook*. Oxford: Oxford University Press.

APPENDIX 3: FAMILY PLANNING AND CONTRACEPTION IN GENERAL PRACTICE: GUIDANCE FOR NURSES

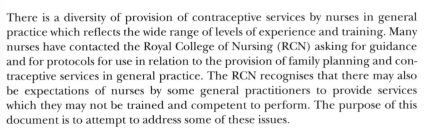

- ❖ **Education**
- ❖ **Protocols**
- ❖ **Prescribing and supply**
- ❖ **Professional accountability**
- ❖ **Recommendations**
- ❖ **References**

There is a diversity of provision of contraceptive services by nurses in general practice which reflects the wide range of levels of experience and training. Many nurses have contacted the Royal College of Nursing (RCN) asking for guidance and for protocols for use in relation to the provision of family planning and contraceptive services in general practice. The RCN recognises that there may also be expectations of nurses by some general practitioners to provide services which they may not be trained and competent to perform. The purpose of this document is to attempt to address some of these issues.

EDUCATION

There are courses available in all four countries that have been approved by the respective National Boards. The National Boards produce an outline syllabus, but the format and educational level varies across the United Kingdom. The courses are run by colleges and universities and are regularly reviewed. Future developments will allow access to modular courses based on prior learning and individual needs and those that lead to a recordable qualification will meet the new requirements for specialist practice (UKCC 1994).

Currently, there are three categories of training available:

❖ Introduction to Family Planning/Sexual Health or Family Planning Appreciation courses. These courses may be organised by colleges, universities or Health Commissions and, therefore, will be accredited accordingly. These courses have no clinical component. They give nurses a basic knowledge of the different methods of contraception and sexual health services available and the mechanisms for appropriate referral. They do not enable nurses to give any clinical care.

❖ ENB 901: Family Planning in Society or the equivalent in Scotland, Northern Ireland and Wales. The courses combine theoretical and practical components – including a clinical assessment – which lead to a certificate of competence. These courses give nurses an in-depth knowledge of all methods of contraception, enabling them to deliver competent clinical care. Although cervical screening is included in the syllabus, not all courses train nurses to take cervical smears. Those that do may not assess competence.

❖ ENB A08: Advanced Family Planning Nursing. This course is becoming more widely available and allows experienced family planning nurses to develop individual specialist skills.

There are a variety of study days and courses specifically designed for qualified family planning nurses to update and maintain their skills and knowledge. They also prepare practitioners to act as supervisors/assessors.

PROTOCOLS

The RCN believes that protocols are valuable tools that should be used. They are derived from practice policies and offer guidance on particular aspects of patient care – for individuals and teams. They help to identify members of the Primary Health Care Team who can work within the protocol.

A protocol is a document which should be individually negotiated between the nurse and her GP/employer. It is not appropriate to use protocols that have been developed by other practitioners.

When producing a protocol consideration should be given to:

❖ the law
❖ the nurse's training, experience and competence
❖ the specific needs of the practice population
❖ the expectations of the GP/employer.

The document should specify:

❖ which activities can be undertaken and by whom, in what circumstances: this may include a written procedure or 'check list'
❖ referral criteria.

PRESCRIBING AND SUPPLY

The use of protocols to facilitate the supply of medicines is under debate with differing legal interpretations of the 1968 Medicines Act and associated legislation. It is acceptable for protocols to be used by appropriately educated and competent family planning nurses for the provision of supply of hormonal contraceptives where the initial assessment and prescription has been made by a doctor and a protocol covering further supply has been drawn up and signed by that doctor, either at the time of consultation or in advance of anticipated follow-up visits.

PROFESSIONAL ACCOUNTABILITY

The UKCC Code of Professional Conduct states that 'as a registered nurse, midwife or health visitor, you are personally accountable for your practice'. All clauses within the code are relevant but those most pertinent are clauses 3 and 4:

(3) *'maintain and improve your professional knowledge and competence'*

(4) *'acknowledge any limitations in your knowledge and competance and decline any duties or responsibilities unless able to perform them in a safe and skilled manner'.*

The UKCC Scope of Professional Practice endorses the above and suggests that if a registered practitioner is aware of her/his professional accountability, and is competent and capable to carry out an activity and that this meets the needs and is in the interests of clients/patients, then a nurse can expand her/his scope of practice as necessary. Therefore, under no circumstances should a nurse, midwife or health visitor undertake a procedure unless she/he is competent to do so. It is the responsibility of the individual nurse to inform her/his manager if they have not had appropriate training.

The ENB issued a 'Dear Colleague' letter in 1993 which clearly states that: 'Those nurses/midwives responsible for direct care in the Family Planning Service within General Practice must undertake the full course.' It also states that nurses working in general practice, who are responsible for answering general queries, must undertake the most appropriate module to meet their needs.

RECOMMENDATIONS

The RCN recommends that:

❖ all nurses working in general practice should attend an 'Introduction to Family Planning' or a Family Planning Appreciation course

❖ at least one nurse in each practice should complete an approved family planning course

❖ each practice should have access to a clinical nurse specialist in family planning in their locality for support and systems of clinical supervision

Appendix 3: RCN Guidelines

❖ all family planning trained nurses must regularly update their knowledge and skills to maintain competence to practice

❖ no nurse working in general practice should undertake family planning advice or clinical care unless she has received the appropriate training.

REFERENCES

Department of Health (1989) *Report of the Advisory Group on Nurse Prescribing.* London: HMSO.

English National Board for Nursing, Midwifery and Health Visiting (1992) *Family Planning in Society. Course Number 901.* London: ENB.

English National Board for Nursing, Midwifery and Health Visiting (1993) *Dear Colleague Letter.* London: ENB.

Scottish National Board for Nursing, Midwifery and Health Visiting – *Family Planning Course.*

Northern Ireland National Board for Nursing, Midwifery and Health Visiting – *Family Planning Course.*

Parliament. *Medicines Act* (1968). London: HMSO.

United Kingdom Central Council for Nursing, Midwifery and Health Visiting (1992) *Code of Professional Conduct.* London: UKCC.

United Kingdom Central Council for Nursing, Midwifery and Health Visiting (1992) *The Scope of Professional Practice.* London: UKCC.

United Kingdom Central Council for Nursing, Midwifery and Health Visiting (1992) *Standards for the Administration of Medicines.* London: UKCC.

Welsh National Board for Nursing, Midwifery and Health Visiting – *WNB 901.*

Published by the Royal College of Nursing, 20 Cavendish Square, London, W1M 0AB. Telephone 0171 409 3333.

First published October 1996 (ref NPC/06/96)

Reorder number 000 631

APPENDIX 4: BREAST PALPATION AND BREAST AWARENESS: GUIDELINES FOR PRACTICE

❖ **The role of the nurse**
❖ **Professional accountability**
❖ **Conclusion**
❖ **References**

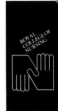

There is currently a diversity of practice among nurses in the UK in the use of breast palpation for health screening or following a diagnosis of breast cancer.

We recognise the concerns and pressures that nurses are under to relieve anxieties when dealing with women with breast problems, be this in primary health care or a hospital setting.

It is acknowledged that the diagnosis of breast cancer is frequently a complex process, best performed by a specialist multi-disciplinary team (King's Fund Forum 1986) involving the combined use of clinical examination (palpation), radiology, pathology and surgery.

It is recognised that even in the most skilled hands the sensitivity and specificity of some diagnostic measures, for example mammography, falls short of 100 per cent (Cancer Research Campaign 1988, DHSS 1986). There is no evidence that palpation alone of the breasts is effective in reducing mortality from breast cancer and it has a lower sensitivity as a diagnostic measure than mammography (DHSS 1986). It should be noted that the Medical and Dental Defence Union of Scotland, in 1992, issued guidelines to general practitioners stating 'We do not recommend that breast palpation is done by practice nurses' (Medical and Dental Defence Union of Scotland 1992).

THE ROLE OF THE NURSE

The nurse's role is to educate and facilitate within this area of health care and to provide information and support for women: it is not to provide a diagnosis or to imply that the nurses can in any way define whether a woman may or may not have breast cancer.

However, it is recommended that nurses promote 'breast awareness' as described within the National Health Service Breast Screening Programme information leaflet (NHSBSP 1994). This should be a part of general body awareness, promoting the process of a woman getting to know her own breasts and becoming familiar with what is normal for her, and thus enabling her to detect the abnormal. In the context of becoming familiar with her breasts a woman may seek the help of a nurse to demonstrate how this might be achieved. This is not breast examination or palpation and this fact should be made clear to the woman. Both verbal and written explanation of what changes to look out for should be given, and most importantly support to the woman to report any such changes. In addition, women should be informed of the availability of routine mammographic breast screening for those over the age of 50 years within the National Health Service Breast Screening Programme and supported should they wish to participate in this.

In the case of particular client groups, for example adults with learning disabilities where the responsibility for breast awareness may of necessity have to rest more with the carer than with the client herself, nurses may need to look for, and report, relevant breast changes in clients and may also need to educate other carers involved with these clients in this area of care. Women from these client groups should also be assisted to participate in the National Health Service Breast Screening Programme.

It should be noted that 1 in 100 cases of breast cancer occur in men.

PROFESSIONAL ACCOUNTABILITY

The UKCC Code of Professional Conduct (UKCC 1992) states that the nurse should:

❖ act always in such a manner as to promote and safeguard the interests and well-being of patients and clients

❖ ensure that no action or omission on your part, or within your sphere of responsibility, is detrimental

❖ acknowledge any limitations in your knowledge and competence and decline any duties or responsibilities unless able to perform them in a safe and skilled manner.

The UKCC Scope of Professional Practice states:

❖ From the point of registration, each practitioner is subject to the Council's Code of Professional Conduct and accountability for his or her practice and conduct

❖ Once registered, each nurse, midwife and health visitor remains subject to the Code and ultimately accountable to the Council for his or her actions and omissions.

In the light of these statements it is clear that nurses are accountable for their individual actions. They therefore should be aware of their responsibilities to the patients and of the legal implications that the practice of breast palpation by a nurse might have, such as litigation for false negative diagnosis.

CONCLUSION

We recommend that nurses do not undertake the practice of breast palpation and if requested to do so within their sphere of practice they should be supported in challenging such 'instruction'.

However, it should be acknowledged that a small number of nurses with specialist training include breast palpation as a significant part of their role. This should only be undertaken within an environment providing immediate on site access to the facilities necessary for the complex process of breast cancer diagnosis.

Appendix 4: RCN Guidelines

REFERENCES

Cancer Research Campaign (1988) *Breast Screening* Factsheet 7.2.

Department of Health and Social Security (1986) *The Forrest Report: Breast Screening* London: HMSO.

King's Fund Forum (1986) Consensus Development Conference. Treatment of Primary Breast Cancer. *British Medical Journal* Vol. 293 pp 946–7.

Medical and Dental Defence Union of Scotland (1992) *Summons* March 1992 pp 1.3.

National Health Service Breast Screening Programme (NHSBSP) 'Be Breast Aware' (1994), prepared by Cancer Research Campaign. London: Department of Health/HMSO.

United Kingdom Central Council for Nursing, Midwifery and Health Visiting (1992) *The Scope of Professional Practice* (paras 4, 5 and 6) London: UKCC.

Published by the Royal College of Nursing, 20 Cavendish Square, London, W1M 0AB. Telephone 0171 409 3333.

First published September 1996 (ref NPC/12/94)

Re-order number 000 552

APPENDIX 5: BIMANUAL PELVIC EXAMINATION: GUIDANCE FOR NURSES

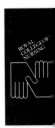

- ❖ **Background**
- ❖ **Bimanual pelvic examination as a screening test for ovarian cancer**
- ❖ **Bimanual pelvic examination in symptomatic women**
- ❖ **Professional accountability**
- ❖ **Recommendation**
- ❖ **Bibliography**

This position statement has been written to clarify the nurses' role in relation to performing a bimanual pelvic examination.

Previous guidance was issued by the Royal College of Nursing (Issues in Nursing and Health: Cervical Screening Guidelines for Good Practice 1994) relating to the taking of a cervical smear. During the course of writing this guidance it became apparent that there was great diversity of practice around the UK about whether a woman had a bimanual pelvic examination performed routinely at the same time as her cervical smear was taken.

Many nurses have contacted the RCN in relation to this issue and also in relation to their concern about the type of training a nurse requires to ensure competency in the bimanual pelvic examination.

BACKGROUND

Controversy exists about the usefulness of routine bimanual pelvic examinations in asymptomatic women when attending for cervical smear. If a woman has no symptoms whatsoever, a bimanual pelvic examination is unlikely to pick up a pathological condition and the examination should therefore not be performed. Endometriosis is unlikely to be picked up on routine bimanual pelvic examination and there is no value in detecting asymptomatic fibroids or benign cysts. If fibroids are important, for example if the woman is symptomatic or is about to start on hormone replacement therapy (HRT), this represents a clinical indication for performing a bimanual pelvic examination. Therefore the key issue is whether there is evidence to support the efficacy of bimanual pelvic examination as a screening test for ovarian cancer.

It is essential that anyone taking a cervical smear has been taught how to locate the cervix, although they will not necessarily know how to do a bimanual pelvic examination. When women do present for a cervical smear it is very important to have a checklist of questions to exclude any under-lying possible pathology, for example the detection of pelvic inflammatory disease (PID). Women are not always aware of the symptoms they should be looking out for and therefore the positive effects of reminding them by direct questions is extremely important. These questions should include:

❖ abdominal swelling?

❖ intermenstrual bleeding?

❖ very painful and/or heavy periods?

❖ lower abdominal pain or discomfort?

❖ post coital bleeding?

❖ pain on intercourse?

❖ urinary symptoms?

Women who have any of these symptoms or signs should have a bimanual pelvic examination by a doctor or nurse who has been appropriately trained.

BIMANUAL PELVIC EXAMINATION AS A SCREENING TEST FOR OVARIAN CANCER

Ovarian cancer is the fifth commonest cancer in women with over 5830 new cases occurring in the UK in 1988 (Cancer Research Campaign 1994).

90% of cases occur in women over 45 years. Because of the lack of early symptoms 65–75% of cases present with advanced disease and the prognosis is poor. In 1992 4360 women died from ovarian cancer in the UK.

When used on its own, bimanual pelvic examination is not a reliable test to detect ovarian cancer. It cannot reliably distinguish between benign and malignant ovarian cysts and there is a high false positive rate detected due to benign disease. Unpublished evidence suggests that the false positive rate is high when bimanual pelvic examinations are performed by a gynaecologist but even higher when performed by GPs and practice nurses (Ian Jacobs, personal communication). The false positive rate is particularly high for premenopausal women.

In the absence of convincing evidence that benign ovarian cysts have malignant potential, bimanual pelvic examination alone is not acceptable as a screening test for ovarian cancer.

The precise sensitivity of pelvic examination is not known. However in two ultrasound studies in Sweden, four of the 10 ovarian cancers detected by ultrasound had negative findings on vaginal examination (Andolf et al (1986), Andolf et al (1990)). In the Kings' College Hospital study, only one of the five primary ovarian cancers could be detected by manual examination after ultrasonography (Campbell et al (1989)).

An additional factor which needs to be taken into account is the acceptability of the bimanual pelvic screening test to the population. The poor uptake which would accompany a test which is not widely acceptable would nullify the benefits of screening. While no specific analysis has been conducted of the acceptability of bimanual pelvic examination, the available evidence suggests that it may be largely unacceptable, particularly to asymptomatic postmenopausal women, yet it is this group who are most at risk of ovarian cancer (UKCCCR (1989)).

BIMANUAL PELVIC EXAMINATION IN SYMPTOMATIC WOMEN

Bimanual pelvic examination should be used to assess symptomatic women and in other cases where clinically indicated. Performing this examination requires expertise and it is absolutely essential that those who undertake such examinations should receive appropriate training and perform sufficient examinations each year to retain their skills.

Recognised screening courses such as Marie Curie Course, the ENB N28 (women's screening and health promotion) and the A08 (advanced family planning course) have a component within them to teach bimanual pelvic examination.

PROFESSIONAL ACCOUNTABILITY

The UKCC Code of Professional Conduct states '. . . As a registered nurse, midwife or health visitor, you are personally accountable for your practice'. All clauses within the code are relevant but those most pertinent are clauses 3 and 4:

(3) 'maintain and improve your professional knowledge and competence'.

(4) 'acknowledge any limitations in your knowledge and competence and decline any duties or responsibilities unless able to perform them in a safe and skilled manner'.

The UKCC Scope of Professional Practice endorses the above and lays professional accountability on the individual practitioner. Therefore under no circumstances should a nurse, midwife or health visitor undertake a procedure unless he/she is competent to do so. It is the responsibility of the individual nurse to inform his/her manager if they have not had appropriate training.

RECOMMENDATION

On the basis of all the evidence currently available, the Bimanual Pelvic Working Group of the RCN and the NHS Cervical Screening Programme National Co-ordinating Network recommends that bimanual pelvic examination should not be undertaken as a routine screening procedure performed on asymptomatic women. Its use in symptomatic women, or in other circumstances where it is clinically indicated, should be restricted to those who have received the appropriate training.

BIBLIOGRAPHY

Andolf E, Svalenius E, Astedt B (1986) Ultrasonography for early detection of ovarian carcinoma. *British Journal of Obstetrics Gynaecology* 93: 1286–9.

Andolf E, Jorgensen C, Astedt B (1990) Ultrasound examination for detection of ovarian carcinoma in risk groups. *British Journal of Obstetrics Gynaecology* 75: 106–9.

Austoker J. (1994) Screening for ovarian, prostatic and testicular cancers. BMJ 309, July, 315–320.

Bourne T, Campbell S, Steer C et al (1989) Transvaginal colour flow imaging: a possible new screening technique for ovarian cancer. BMJ 299: 1367–79.

Campbell S, Bhan V, Royston P et al (1989) Transabdominal ultrasound screening for early ovarian cancer. BMJ 299: 1363–7.

Campbell S et al (1992) Role of colour Doppler in an ultrasound-based screening programme. In Sharp F et al (eds). *Ovarian Cancer. Biology, Diagnosis and Management* pp 237–47 London: Chapman and Hall Medical.

Cancer Research Campaign (1991) Ovarian cancer screening. Factsheet 17.

Cancer Research Campaign (1994) Scientific Yearbook 1994–95.

Collins W et al (1992) Ultrasound for early cancer screening. In F Sharp et al (eds). *Ovarian Cancer. Biology, Diagnosis and Management* pp 225–36 London: Chapman and Hall Medical.

Cuckle H, Wald N (1991) Screening for ovarian cancer. In AB Miller et al (eds), Cancer Screening, pp 228–39 Cambridge University Press and UICC.

Davies A, Oram D, Jacobs I (1991) Tumour markets in screening for ovarian cancer. In AB Miller et al (eds), Cancer Screening, pp 205–20 Cambridge University Press and UICC.

Dembo A, Davy M, Stenwig A et al (1990) Prognostic factors in patients with stage one epithelial ovarian cancer, 263–73 *British Journal of Obstetrics Gynaecology 75.*

Jacobs I, Stabile I, Bridges J et al (1988) Multimodal approach to screening for ovarian cancer. *Lancet* i: 268–71.

Jacobs I, Bast R (1989) The CA 125 tumour-associated antigen: a review of the literature. *Human Reprod* 4: 1–12.

Jacobs I, Oram D (1990) Potential screening tests for ovarian cancer. In Sharp F et al (eds) *Ovarian Cancer, Biological and Therapeutic Challenges* pp 197–205 London: Chapman and Hall Medical.

Jacobs I, Prys Davies A, Bridges J et al (1993) Prevalence of screening for ovarian cancer in postmenopausal women by CA 125 measurement and ultrasonography. BMJ 306: 1030–4.

Jacobs I, Prys Davies A, Oram D (1992) Role of CA 125 in screening for ovarian cancer. In F Sharp et al (eds). *Ovarian Cancer, Biology, Diagnosis and Management* pp 265–73 London: Chapman and Hall Medical.

Jacobs I (1994) Screening for epithelial ovarian cancer. *Lancet* 343: 337–8.

Royal College of Nursing (1994) *Issues in Health* No. 28. Cervical Screening Guidelines for Good Practice. London: RCN.

Scott I (1992) Advantages and disadvantages of randomized controlled trials of ovarian cancer screening. In Sharp F et al (eds). *Ovarian Cancer. Biology, Diagnosis and Management* pp 277–87 London: Chapman and Hall Medical.

Smith L, Ol R (1984) Detection of malignant ovarian neoplasms: a review of the literature. 2. Laboratory detection. 3. Immunological detection and ovarian cancer-associated antigens. *British Journal of Obstetrics Gynaecology Survey* 39: 329–45, 346–60.

UKCC (1992) Code of Professional Conduct. London: UKCC.

UKCC (1992) The Scope of Professional Practice. London: UKCC.

UKCCCR (1989) Ovarian Cancer Screening (Report). (UKCCCR, London).

Wald N, Parkes C (1993) Screening for ovarian cancer. BMJ 306: 1684.

Webb M (1993) Screening for ovarian cancer. BMJ 306: 1015–6.

Published by the Royal College of Nursing, 20 Cavendish Square, London W1M 0AB. Telephone 0171 409 3333.

Re-order number 000 528

REFERENCES

Albert, A.E., Warner, D.L., Hatcher, R.A., Trussell, J. & Bennett, C. (1995) Condom use among female commercial sex workers in Nevada's legal brothels. *American Journal of Public Health* **85:**1514–1520.

Allen, M.E. (ed.) (1991) *Good Clinical Practice in Europe. Investigator's Handbook*, pp. 19–35. Romford: Rostrum Publications.

Allison, C.J. (1995) Long term use of Nova T intrauterine device beyond five years compared with routine refitting after five years of use: a multicentre study. *British Journal of Family Planning* **21:**82–84.

Andersson, K., Mattsson, L-M., Rybo, G. & Stadberg, E. (1992) Intrauterine release of levonorgestrel – a new way of adding progestogen in hormone replacement therapy. *Obstetrics and Gynaecology* **79:**963–967.

Andersson, K., Odlind, V. & Rybo, G. (1994) Levonorgestrel-releasing and copper releasing (Nova T) IUDs during five years of use: A randomised comparative trial. *Contraception* **49:**56–72.

Bagwell, M.A., Coker, A.L., Thompson, S.J., Baker, E.R. & Addy, C.L. (1995) Primary infertility and oral contraceptive steroid use. *Fertility and Sterility* **63:**1161–1166.

Balen, A., Challis, J., West, C., Valentine, A. & Steele, S.J. (1994) A survey of dietary awareness in women who are planning a pregnancy. *The British Journal of Family Planning* **20:**96.

Belfield, T. (1997) *FPA Contraceptive Handbook*, 2nd edition. London: Family Planning Association (FPA).

Bird, K.D. (1991) The use of spermicide containing nonoxynol-9 in the prevention of HIV infection. *Aids* **5:**791–796.

Birth Control Trust (1994) Briefing: possible association between abortion and breast cancer. *Letter.*

Blain, S., Oloto, E., Meyrick, I. & Bromham, D. (1996) Skin reactions following Norplant insertion and removal – possible causative factors. *The British Journal of Family Planning* **21:**130–132.

BMA, GMSC, HEA, Brook Advisory Centres, FPA & RCGP (1993) Joint guidance note: *Confidentiality and People Under 16*. British Medical Association, General Medical Science Committee, Health Education Authority, Brook Advisory Centres, Family Planning Association and Royal College of General Practitioners.

Bonn, D. (1996) What prospects for hormonal contraceptives for men? *The Lancet* **347:**316.

Bontis, J., Vavilis, D., Theodoridis, T. & Sidropoulou, A. (1994) Copper intrauterine contraceptive device and pregnancy rate. *Advances in Contraception* **10:**205–211.

Bounds, W. (1994) Contraceptive efficacy of the diaphragm and cervical caps used in conjunction with a spermicide – a fresh look at the evidence. *The British Journal of Family Planning* **20**:84–87.

Bounds, W., Kubba, A., Tayob, Y., Mills, A. & Guillebaud, J. (1986) Clinical trial of a spermicide-free, custom-fitted, valued cervical cap (Contracap). *British Journal of Family Planning* **11**:125–131.

Bounds, W., Guillebaud, J. & Newman, G.B. (1992a) Female condom (Femidom). A clinical study of its use-effectiveness and patient acceptability. *The British Journal of Family Planning* **18**:36–41.

Bounds, W., Hutt, S., Kubba, A., Cooper, K., Guillebaud, J. & Newman, G.B. (1992b) Randomised comparative study in 217 women of three disposable plastic IUCD thread retrievers. *British Journal of Obstetrics and Gynaecology* **99**:915–919.

Bounds, W., Robinson, G., Kubba, A. & Guillebaud, J. (1993) Clinical experience with a levonorgestrel-releasing intrauterine contraceptive device (LNG-IUD) as a contraceptive and in the treatment of menorrhagia. *The British Journal of Family Planning* **19**:193–194.

Bounds, W., Guillebaud, J., Dominik, R. & Dalberth, B. (1995) The diaphragm with and without spermicide. A randomised, comparative efficacy trial. *The Journal of Reproductive Medicine* **40**:764–774.

Brahams, D. (1995) Medicine and the law: Warning about natural reversal of vasectomy. *The Lancet* **345**:444.

Bromham, D.R. (1996) Contraceptive implants. *British Medical Journal* **312**:1555–1556.

Canter, A.K. & Goldthorpe, S.B. (1995), Vasectomy – patient satisfaction in general practice: A follow up study. *The British Journal of Family Planning* **21**:58–60.

Cardy, G.C. (1995) Outcome of pregnancies after failed hormonal postcoital contraception – an interim report. *The British Journal of Family Planning* **21**:112–115.

Cayley, J. (1995) Emergency contraception – time to loosen medical controls over its availability. *British Medical Journal* **311**:762–763.

Chantler, E. (1992) Vaginal spermicides: some current concerns. *British Journal of Family Planning* **17**: 118–119.

Chilvers, C. (1994) Breast cancer and depot-medroxyprogesterone acetate: A review. *Contraception* **49**: 211–222.

Clubb, E. & Knight, J. (1996) *Fertility*. Newton Abbot: David & Charles.

Collaborative Group on Hormonal Factors in Breast Cancer (1996) Breast cancer and hormonal contraceptives: Collaborative reanalysis of individual data on 53 297 women with breast cancer and 100 239 woman without breast cancer from 54 epidemiological studies. *The Lancet* **347**:1713–1727.

Collaborative Group on Hormonal Factors in Breast Cancer (1996) Breast cancer and hormonal contraceptives. *Contraception* **54**:3 (supplement).

Conor, S. & Kingman, S. (1988) *The Search for the Virus. The Discovery of AIDS and the Quest for a Cure*. London: Penguin Books.

Coutinho, E.M., De Souza, J.C., Athayde, C., Barbosa, I.C., Alvarez, F., Brache, V., Zhi-Ping, G., Emuveyan, E.E., Adeyemi, O., Devoto, L., Shaabam, M.M., Salem, H.T., Affandi, B., Mateo de Accosta, O., Mati, J. & Ladipo, O.A. (1996) Multi centre clinical trial on the efficacy and acceptability of a single contraceptive implant of Normegestrol Acetate, Uniplant. *Contraception* **53**:121–125.

Cresswell, J.L. (1996) Foetal and infant origins of adult disease. *Hospital Update* **116:**120–126.

Crosier, A. (1996) Women's knowledge and awareness of emergency contraception. *The British Journal of Family Planning* **22:**87–90.

CSAC (1993a) Long term progestogen only contraception (injection and oral) and effect on oestrogen. *British Journal of Family Planning* **18:**134–135.

CSAC (1993b) Retention of IUDs after the menopause. *British Journal of Family Planning* **18:**134–135.

Cushman, L.F., Davidson, A.R., Kalmuss, D., Heartwell, S. & Rulin, M. (1996) Beliefs about Norplant Implants among low income urban women. *Contraception* **53:**285–291.

Cundy, T., Evans, M., Roberts, H., Wattie, D., Ames, R. & Reid, I.R. (1991) Bone density in women receiving depot medroxyprogesterone acetate for contraception. *British Medical Journal* **303:**13–16.

Cundy, T., Cornish, J., Evans, M.C., Roberts, H. & Reid, I.R. (1994) Recovery of bone density in women who stop using medroxyprogesterone acetate. *British Medical Journal* **308:**247–248.

Dalton, K. (1983) *Once a Month.* Glasgow: Fontana.

Darney, P., Klaisle, C.M., Tanner, S. & Alvarado, A.M. (1990) Sustained release contraceptives. *Current Problems in Obstetrics, Gynaecology and Fertility* **13:** 99–100.

Davidson, J.A.H. (1992) Warming lignocaine to reduce pain associated with injection. *British Medical Journal* **305:**617–618.

de Jong, F.H. (1987) Inhibin – its nature, site of production and function. In Clarke, J.R. (ed.) *Oxford Review of Reproductive Biology*, Vol. 9. Oxford: Oxford University Press.

Department of Health (1992a) *The Health of the Nation: A summary of the strategy for health in England.* London: HMSO:22.

Department of Health (1992b) *Folic Acid and Neural Tube Defects: Guidelines on Prevention.* London: Department of Health (*Letter*).

Department of Health (1992c) *Immunisation against Infectious Disease.* London: HMSO:68.

Department of Health (1995) The response for doctors to the Committee on Safety of Medicines letter. *FPA & Faculty of Family Planning and Reproductive Health Care of the Royal College of Obstetricians & Gynaecologists.*

Diaz, J., Faundes, A., Olmos, P. & Diaz, M. (1996) Bleeding complaints during the first year of Norplant implants use and their impact on removal rate. *Contraception* **53:**91–95.

Drug and Therapeutics Bulletin (1996a) Topiramate – add on drug for partial seizures. *Drug and Therapeutics Bulletin* **34:**62–64.

Drug and Therapeutics Bulletin (1996b). Hormone replacement therapy. *Drug and Therapeutics Bulletin* **34:**81–84.

Durex (1993) *History of the condom.* London: Durex Information Service.

Durex (1994) The Durex report 1994: a summary of consumer research into contraception. London: Durex Information Service.

Editorial (1996) Pill scares and public responsibility. *The Lancet* **347:**1707.

Faculty of Family Planning and Reproductive Health Care of the Royal College of Obstetricians and Gynaecologists (1996) Statement on hormonal contraceptives and breast cancer, Thursday 20 June 1996, (*Letter*).

References

Farley, T.M.M., Rosenberg, M.J., Rowe, P.J., Chen, J-H. & Meirik, O. (1992) Intrauterine devices and pelvic inflammatory disease: An international perspective. *The Lancet* **339:**785–788.

Farr, G. & Amatya, R. (1994) Contraception and efficacy of the copper T 380A and copper T 200 intrauterine devices: Results from a comparative clinical trial in six developing countries. *Contraception* **49:**231–243.

Farr, G., Amatya, R., Doh, A., Ekwempu, C.C., Toppozada, M. & Ruminjo, J. (1996) An evaluation of the copper–T 380A IUD's safety and efficacy at three African centers. *Contraception* **53:**293–298.

Flynn, A. (1996). Natural family planning. *The British Journal of Family Planning* **21:**146–148.

Ford, N. & Mathie, E. (1993) The acceptability and experience of the female condom, Femidom among family planning clinic attenders. *The British Journal of Family Planning* **19:**187–192.

Fowler, P. (1996) Subdermal implants – still a viable long-term contraceptive option? *The British Journal of Family Planning* **22:**31–33.

FPA (1993) *Vasectomy and Prostrate Cancer.* London: Family Planning Association.

FPA (1995) FPA Fact file 3B: *Contraception: Some Factors Affecting Research and Development.* London: Family Planning Association.

Gillmer, M.D., Walling, M.R. & Povey, S.J. (1996) The effect on serum lipids and lipoproteins of three combined oral contraceptives containing norgestimate, gestodene and desogestrel. *The British Journal of Family Planning* **22:**67–71.

Giovannucci, E., Ascherio, A., Rimm, E., Colditz, G.A., Stampfer, M.J. & Wilett, W.C. (1993a) A prospective cohort study of vasectomy and prostate cancer in US men. *Journal of the American Medical Association* **269:** 873–877.

Giovannucci, E., Tosteson, T.D., Speizer, F.E., Ascherio, A., Vessey, M.P. & Colditz, G.A. (1993b) A retrospective cohort study of vasectomy and prostate cancer in US men. *Journal of the America Medical Association* **269:** 878–882.

Goldbeck-Wood, S. (1994) Researchers claim abortion increases risk of breast cancer. *British Medical Journal* **313:** 962.

Gooder, P. (1996) Knowledge of emergency contraception amongst men and women in the general population and women seeking an abortion. *The British Journal of Family Planning* **22:**81–84.

Grady, W.R., Klepinger, D.H., Billy, J.O.G. & Tanfer, K. (1993) Condom characteristics: The perceptions and preferences of men in the United States. *Family Planning Perspective* **25:**67–73.

Guillebaud J. (1993) *Contraception: Your Questions Answered,* 2nd edition. Edinburgh: Churchill Livingstone.

Guillebaud, J. (1995) *Contraception Today.* London: Martin Dunitz Limited.

Guillebaud, J. (1997) *Contraception Today,* 3rd edition. London: Martin Dunitz Limited.

Guillebaud, J. & Bounds, W. (1983) Control of pain associated with intrauterine device insertion using mefenamic acid. *Research and Clinical Forums* **5:**69–74.

Ho, P.C. & Kwan, M.S.W. (1993) A prospective randomised comparison of levonorgestrel with the Yuzpe regimen in post-coital contraception. *Human Reproduction* **8:**389–392.

Hollingworth, B. & Guillebaud, J. (1994) The levonorgestrel intrauterine device. *The Diplomate* **1:**247–251.

House of Commons Health Committee (1990–91) *Maternity Services: Preconception.* London: HMSO (Fourth report, Vol. 1).

Howards, S.S. & Peterson, H.B. (1993) Vasectomy and prostate cancer. Chance, bias or a causal relationship. *Journal of the American Medical Association* **269:** 913–914.

Hudson, G. & Hawkins, R. (1995) Contraception practices of women attending for termination of pregnancy – a study from South Australia. *The British Journal of Family Planning* **21:**61–64.

Hughes, H. & Myers, P. (1996) Women's knowledge and preference about emergency contraception: A survey from a rural general practice. *The British Journal of Family Planning* **22:**77–78.

Indian Council of Medical Research Task Force on Natural Family Planning (1996) Field trial of Billings ovulation method of natural family planning. *Contraception* **53:**69–74.

International Family Planning Perspectives (1992) Invasive cervical cancer risk no greater for DMPA users than for nonusers. *International Family Planning Perspectives.* **18:**156–157.

Jick, H., Jick, S.S., Gurewich, V., Myers, M.W. & Vasilakis, C. (1995) Risk of idiopathic cardiovascular death and nonfatal venous thromboembolism in women using oral contraceptives with differing progestagen components. *The Lancet* **346:**1589–1592.

Kubba, A. (1995) *Emergency Contraception Guidelines for Doctors.* Faculty of Family Planning and Reproductive Health Care of the RCOG.

Leiras (1995) Mirena levonorgestrel 20 micrograms/24 hours. Product monograph. Finland: Leiras.

Lewis, M.A., Spitzer, W.O., Heinemann, L.A.J., Macrae, K.D., Bruppacher, R. & Thorogood, M. (1996) Third generation oral contraceptives and risk of myocardial infarction: An international case control study. *British Medical Journal* **312:**88–90.

Luukkainen, T. (1993) The levonorgestrel releasing IUD. *British Journal of Family Planning* **19:**221–224.

McCann, M.F. & Potter, L.S. (1994) Progestin-only oral contraception: A comprehensive review. *Contraception* **50:**S3–S195.

McEwan, H. (1990) The menopause. In Pfeffer, N. & Quick, A. (eds) *Promoting Women's Health.* London: King Edward's Hospital Fund for London.

Machin, S.J., Mackie, I.J. & Guillebaud, J. (1995) Factor V Leiden mutation, venous thromboembolism and combined oral contraceptive usage. *British Journal of Family Planning* **21:**13–14.

Mascarenhas, L., Newton, P. & Newton, J. (1994) First clinical experience with contraceptive implants in the U.K. *British Journal of Family Planning* **20:**60 (*Letter*).

Mishell, D.R. (ed.) (1994) Papers presented at a World Health Organisation meeting on Once-a-month combined injectable contraception – Part 1. *Contraception* **49:**291–420.

National Institutes of Health (1993) Final statement – March 2, 1993. Vasectomy and prostate cancer conference USA. Family Health International. Bethseda, Maryland: National Institute of Child Health and Human Development.

Niruthisard, S., Roddy, R. & Chutivongse, S. (1991) The effects of frequent Nonoxynol-9 use on the vaginal and cervical mucosa. *Sexually Transmitted Diseases.* **18:**176–179.

References

OPCS (1991) Office of Population Census and Surveys, *Abortion Statistics England and Wales*. London: *HMSO*. Series AB.18.

Owen Drife, J. (1993) Deregulating emergency contraception – justified on current information. *British Medical Journal* **307**:695–696.

Parkes, A.S. (1976) *Patterns of Sexuality and Reproduction*. Oxford: Oxford University Press.

Pearson, V.A.H., Owen, M.R., Phillips, D.R., Pereira Gray, D.J. & Marshall, M.N. (1995) Pregnant teenagers' knowledge and use of emergency contraception. *British Medical Journal* **310**:1644.

Pisake, L. (1994) Depot-medroxyprogesterone acetate (DMPA) and cancer of the endometrium and ovary. *Contraception* **49**:203–209.

Raudaskoski, T.H., Lahti, E.I., Kauppila, A.J., Apajasarkkinen, M.A. & Laatikainen, T.J. (1995) Transdermal estrogen with a levonorgestrel-releasing intrauterine device for climacteric complaints: Clinical and endometrial responses. *American Journal of Obstetrics and Gynaecology* **172**:114–119.

Robinson, G.E. (1994) Low-dose combined oral contraceptives. *British Journal of Obstetrics and Gynaecology* **101**:1036–1041.

Robinson, G.E., Bounds, W., Kubba, A., Judith, A. & Guillebaud, J. (1989) Functional ovarian cysts associated with the levonorgestrel releasing device. *British Journal of Family Planning* **14**:131–132.

Roddy, R.E., Cordero, M., Cordero, C. & Fortney, J.A. (1993) A dosing study of nonoxynol-9 and genital irritation. *International Journal of STD & AIDS* **4**:165–170.

Roussel Laboratories Ltd (1994) *Norplant Product Review*. London: Haymarket Medical Imprint.

Rulin, M.C., Davidson, A.R., Philliber, S.G., Graves, W.L. & Cushman, L.F. (1993) Long-term effect of tubal sterilization on menstrual indices and pelvic pain. *Obstetrics and Gynaecology* **82**:118–121.

Ruminjo, J.K., Amatya, R.N., Dunson, T.R., Kruegers, S.L & Chi, I.C. (1996) Norplant implants acceptability and user satisfaction among women in two African countries. *Contraception* **53**:101–107.

Ryder, B. & Campbell, H. (1995) Natural family planning in the 1990s. *The Lancet* **346**:233–234.

Saracco, A., Musicco, M., Nicolosi, A., Angarano, G., Arici, C., Gavazzeni, G., Costigliola, P., Gafa, S., Gervasoni, C., Luzzati, R., Piccinino, F., Puppo, F., Turbessi, G., Vigevani, G.M., Visco, G., Zerboni, R. & Lazzarin, A. (1993) Man-to-woman sexual transmission of HIV: Longitudinal study of 343 steady partners of infected men. *Journal of Acquired Immune Deficiency Syndromes* **6**:497–502.

Short, R.A. (1994) Contraceptives of the future in the light of HIV infection. *Australian New Zealand Obstetric Gynaecology* **34**:330–332.

Sivin, I. (1988) International experience with Norplant and Norplant 2 contraceptives. *Studies in Family Planning* **19**:81–94.

Sivin, I. & Stern, J. (1994) Health during use of levonorgestrel 20 µg/d and the copper TCU 380Ag intrauterine contraceptive devices: a multicenter study. *Fertility and Sterility* **61**:70–77.

Sparrow, M.J. & Lavill, K. (1994) Breakage and slippage of condoms in family planning clients. *Contraception* **50**:117–129.

Spitzer, W.O., Lewis, M.A., Heinemann, L.A.J., Thorogood, M. & Macrae, K.D.

(1996) Third generation oral contraceptives and risk of venous thromboembolic disorders: an international case-control study. *British Medical Journal* **312:**83–88.

Stuttaford, T. (1996) An ex-sailor remedy for a wilting libido. *The Times* 17 October, p. 20.

Suhonen, S., Lahteenmaki, P., Haukkamaa, M., Rutanen, E.-M. & Holstrom, T. (1996) Endometrial response to hormone replacement therapy as assessed by expression of insulin-like growth factor-binding protein 1 in the endometrium. *Fertility and Sterility* **65:**776–782.

The Economist (1995) On the needless hounding of a safe contraceptive. Science and technology. *The Economist* 2 September, pp. 113–114.

The Population Council (1990) *Norplant Levonorgestrel Implants: A Summary of Scientific Data.* New York. The Population Council.

Trimmer, E. (1978) *Basic Sexual Medicine.* London: Heinemann Medical.

Trussell, J. & Stewart, F. (1992) The effectiveness of postcoital hormonal contraception. *Family Planning Perspectives* **24:**262–264.

Trussell, J., Sturgen, K., Stickler, J. & Dominik, R. (1994) Comparative contraceptive efficacy of the female condom and other barrier methods. *Family Planning Perspectives* **26:**66–72.

Trussell, J., Ellertson, C. & Stewart, F. (1996) The effectiveness of the Yuzpe regimen of emergency contraception. *Family Planning Perspectives* **28:**58–64, 87.

UK Family Planning Research Network (1993) Mishaps occurring during condom use, and the subsequent use of post-coital contraception. *British Journal of Family Planning* **19:**218–220.

Vessey, M.P. (1988) Urinary tract infection and the diaphragm. *British Journal of Family Planning* **13:**41–43.

Vessey, M.P., Lawless, M., Yeates, D. & McPherson, K. (1985) Progestogen-only oral contraception. Findings in a large prospective study with special reference to effectiveness. *British Journal of Family Planning* **10:**121–126.

Vessey, M.P., Villard-Mackintosh, L. & Yeates, D. (1990) Effectiveness of progestogen only oral contraceptives. *British Journal of Family Planning* **16:**79 (*Letter*).

de Vincenzi, I. (1994) A longitudinal study of human immunodeficiency virus transmission by heterosexual partners. *New England Journal of Medicine* **331:**331, 341–346.

West, R.R. (1992) Vasectomy and testicular cancer – no association on current evidence. *British Medical Journal* **304:**729–730.

WHO (1981) *Research on the Menopause.* World Health Organization Technical Report No. 670. Geneva: WHO.

WHO (1991) World Health Organization Collaborative Study of Neoplasia and Steroid Contraceptives (1991). Breast cancer and depot-medroxyprogesterone acetate: a multinational study. *The Lancet* **338:**833–838.

WHO (1992) World Health Organization Collaborative Study of Neoplasia and Steroid Contraceptives (1992). Depot medroxyprogesterone acetate (DMPA) and risk of invasive squamous cell cervical cancer. *Contraception* **45:**299–312.

WHO (1995) World Health Organization Collaborative Study of Cardiovascular Disease and Steroid Hormone Contraception. Venous thromboembolic disease and combined oral contraceptives: Results of international multicentre case control study. *The Lancet* **346:**1575–1581.

References

Wildemeersch, D., Van Kets, H., Vrijens, M., Van Trappen, Y., Temmerman, M., Batar, I., Barri, P., Martinez, F., Iglesias-Cortit, L. & Thiery, M. (1994) IUD tolerance in nulligravid and parous women: optimal acceptance with the frameless CuFix implant (GyneFix). Long-term results with a new inserter. *British Journal of Family Planning* **20:**2–5.

Wilson, E. (1993) Depoprovera: Underused and undervalued. *British Medical Journal* **18:**101.

Wilson, E.W. & Rennie, P.I.C. (1976) *The Menstrual Cycle.* London: Lloyd-Luke.

Ziebland, S., Maxwell, K. & Greenhall, E. (1996) 'It's a mega dose of hormones, isn't it?' Why women may be reluctant to use emergency contraception. *British Journal of Family Planning* **22:**84–86.

INDEX

Numbers in italic refer to tables or illustrations; numbers in bold (in a string of numbers) refer to main discussion

Index

Index

Index

Index